Supporting Troubled Young People

A practical guide to helping
with mental health problems

In memory of Mary and James Walker and their grandchildren Leigh, Hannah, Dean, Aimee and Rose.

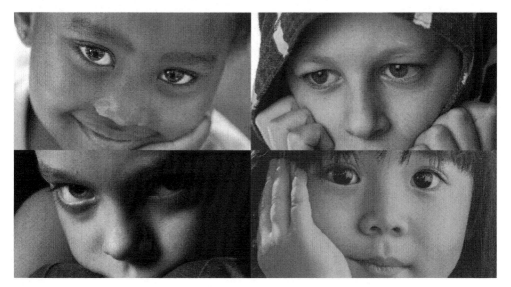

Supporting Troubled Young People

A practical guide to helping with mental health problems

Steven Walker

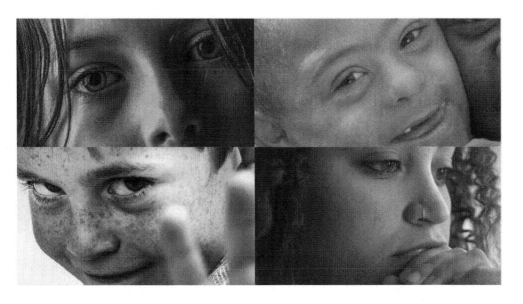

First published in 2019 by Critical Publishing Ltd

British Library Cataloguing in Publication Data
A CIP record for this book is available from the British Library

ISBN: 978-1-912508-73-0

This book is also available in the following e-book formats:
MOBI ISBN: 978-1-912508-74-7
EPUB ISBN: 978-1-912508-75-4
Adobe e-book ISBN: 978-1-912508-76-1

Cover and text design by Out of House Ltd
Project Management by Newgen Publishing UK
Printed and bound in Great Britain by 4edge, Essex

Critical Publishing
3 Connaught Road
St Albans
AL3 5RX

www.criticalpublishing.com

Paper from responsible sources

CONTENTS

MEET THE AUTHOR

Steven Walker was born and raised in a mining community in the north-east of England. A grammar school boy, he is an alumnus of the London School of Economics and Political Science, and has an MPhil in Child and Adolescent Mental Health. He qualified as a psychotherapist in 1992 and worked in CAMHS for 20 years as a practitioner and then Head of Child and Adolescent Mental Health at Anglia Ruskin University, where he designed and developed award-winning multidisciplinary CAMH training. Steven has published 12 textbooks, presented his research at 10 international conferences and published over 50 scholarly papers for international journals.

Steven is a member of the International Family Therapy Association, UK Children and Young People's Mental Health Coalition, International Council of Professional Therapists, and a Volunteer Counsellor with a UK Youth Charity.

This book makes a rich contribution to the understanding and treatment of children's mental health at a time when this is desperately needed. It is well-informed, full of case illustrations to guide the reader, and is written by a compassionate therapist and researcher with a solid grasp of the complex social environment in which children live today.

Dr Chris Nicholson
Head of the Department of Psychosocial and
Psychoanalytic Studies, University of Essex

FOREWORD

Each torpid turn of the world has such disinherited children, to whom no longer what's been, and not yet what's coming, belongs.

These words by the poet Rilke could be written for today's generation of children, children who seem to have been disinherited by an adult society preoccupied with its own concerns and troubles. It was once widely acknowledged that 'the promotion and treatment of children's mental health is everybody's business' (Wilson, 2011). We are now nearly a decade on from this proclamation, but it would seem that the idea of sharing responsibly for children's mental health has been completely forgotten, especially by the UK Government. The 2017 Green Paper for children and young people's mental health services, and promise of parity of esteem of mental health with physical health, has not provided a step-change in the care and treatment of children struggling with adversity and distress. Indeed, every year the NSPCC report a higher frequency of children reporting self-harm through their helpline, while schools and universities are facing a year by year increase in demand for health and wellbeing services, and report of suicide in younger people is a regular signal of concern in the media. Over the same period local resources for children, community and youth services have been cut back and much of the UK's CAMHS provision based upon the IAPT model, are limited to short-term, solution-focused approaches, even for those with acute needs. The original IAPT plan was to improve choice but the result is that fewer models of therapy are on offer. The availability of non-IAPT therapies such as longer-term child psychotherapy for more complex presenting cases is now practically non-existent on the NHS (Mind, 2010). All the while that social and relational capital in local communities is diminishing children have unprecedented access to digital parenting and free run in the cruel virtual playground of social media.

So often we are left with a short term, quick-fix approach to children's mental health which extends conveniently from of a neo-liberal free market economy. In such an approach workers can be quickly trained on mass by power-point to 'deliver' therapy in a series of proscribed steps, never veering from the script to account for actual experiences and the lived difficulties of the child. This approach has been aptly named 'the "McDonaldization" of children's mental health' (Taimimi, 2009) – the therapeutic equivalent of fast-food. Perhaps it is little wonder that some children, not the resilient and the loved, but the disaffected, disenchanted and the dislocated, seem to be lost, disinherited by each torpid turn our society takes.

But the picture is certainly not limited by what I have laid out above. There is a strong alternative approach. All those who come into contact with troubled young people need to be capable of a special form of attention. This form of attention is not reactive, medicalised or procedural, since these kinds of attention are so often defensive. This form of attention starts with a capacity to accept children as they are, to think carefully about them, about the meaning of their behaviour and the possible stresses and influences affecting them; about the acute sense of unease they seem to feel and about the best means of intervening in non-intrusive but helpful ways. It is this kind of attention that Steven Walker's timely book supplies.

Coming in the light of the Government's 2017 Green Paper for children and young people's mental health services, this book has been written as a practical resource for those professionals (teachers, social workers, nurses, youth workers, doctors, foster carers, residential staff, psychologists and psychiatrists) who routinely support and care for young people. Such children need to feel inherited: fully taken on and warmly accepted by professionals who are themselves resilient enough to experience and contain children's distress without becoming contaminated by it, overwhelmed by it or defensively reactive to it. Readers of this book will see the value of such an approach and learn, as they move through each clearly structured chapter, how this approach works.

Walker defines and categorises the main mental health problems and behaviours. He offers useful distinctions between terms such as mental health 'problem', mental health 'disorder' and mental health 'illness'. He details the extent of mental health problems in the UK and the factors involved in the increasing rates seen over the last 10 years. He covers the increase in child poverty, the staggering numbers of children imprisoned in secure institutions and psychiatric units, and the growing rate of cases of gross indecency perpetrated against children. He describes children's experiences of social media, the effects of cyber-bullying and how professional can attend to the issues here without alarmist responses or extreme solutions. As a systemic psychotherapist Walker is well-placed to describe the problematic interactional patterns that can become embedded in family life, and how best to work with the whole family. He has fascinating things to say about research into the role of grandparents.

This book also deals very effectively with issues that were never more important than now, issues of difference, cultural diversity and inclusivity. Children arriving at mental health services may already have experienced exclusion and marginalisation based on prejudicial and outmoded attitudes of those in more powerful positions than themselves. They often carry a feeling of shame and stigma sensing themselves to be somehow 'wrong' in their bodies, and not 'fitting' comfortably with others. However, this primary experience of exclusion is exacerbated by what I will call 'secondary exclusion'. Secondary exclusion occurs when services meant to support children are not in fact sufficiently alert to their needs or when workers lack an appreciation of the specific social factors that have affected their lives until now. It is quite natural that practitioners may sometimes struggle to form an emotional connection with clients who come from different social, intellectual, political or religious backgrounds to themselves. The guidance in this book will be invaluable in helping workers to reflect on this, consider their own subjective experiences and to find a way to approach this honestly. This should ensure that primary exclusion and marginalisation is not repeated and reinforced for young people upon entering services.

We are living in a period when the training offered by an overstretched and underfunded CAMHS is somewhat risk-averse and focused on the technicalities of safeguarding procedures, and digital recording rather than equipping staff to make an essential explorative review of the psychosocial factors contributing to the child's problems, or guiding workers in the tricky process of forming relationships with children who, with good reason, will be suspicious, distrustful and resistant. Steven Walker's book is incredibly helpful in covering the wide range of issues influencing mental health and steps which a thoughtful practitioner would need to take in working with this complexity. Walker covers several broad approaches and their suitability for different mental health disorders, how to undertake a thorough assessment and the ethical issues that arise in developing an effective treatment plan. With great clarity he sets out the legal framework within which practitioners must act, but he also interprets this for the worker by a series of discussions, for example, about competence and children's rights.

This book, broadly speaking, takes a psychosocial approach in which the specificity of children's psychological difficulties are set within, and seen as deeply rooted in, the social, political and familial context. Whilst clearly aware of psychiatric assessment and practice, Walker centres instead upon 'facilitating communication' and thus establishing better social and relational environments around the child. This remind us of Dockar-Drysdale's comment that 'the violent behaviour of a child always means there has been a breakdown in communication' (Dockar-Drysdale 1999). Behaviour is always a communication. It is a communication about the child's emotional state and internal world but also about the familial and social systems they find themselves in. For this reason, Walker also ensures attention is paid not only to the specific presenting problem but also to the environmental factors which naturally have an impact upon this, including how workers from diverse agencies will respond to the same problem very differently (illustrated in Table 7.1). Walker suggests that services have tended to focus their attention on a particular problem. He writes:

For example psychiatric services focus on mental health, drug and alcohol services on drug and alcohol abuse, and pediatric services on physical health. CAMHS guidelines often concentrate on the management of a single mental disorder instead of taking a holistic and co-ordinated approach to care and treatment of the whole person. Too often young people complain that specialist CAMH services focus on their symptoms or diagnostic label and ignore their social needs.

This narrow approach, however, does not reflect the complexity of health problems experienced by children and adolescents, as young people with mental health problems in one area often experience difficulties in other areas of their lives.

There is a sympathy and compassion in his approach which underlines the importance of personal style above process. Here is no empty behavioural rhetoric but rather a thoughtful willingness to meet the child in all their real complexity and aliveness.

Walker comes with a wealth of direct professional experience working with children and their families. As a practitioner-led academic Walker this has always been dedicated to bringing theory together with practice and allowing young people to speak for themselves. I first encountered Steven Walker when he was running an award winning course, Advanced Studies in Child and Adolescence Mental health, at Anglia Ruskin University in Chelmsford. At this time I was supporting a Young Person's Advisory Board run by Colchester MIND. These young people all had experience of diagnosis and treatment in residential psychiatric services. Steven invited them to visit the programme, meet his students and give a presentation, which the young people took very seriously. They spoke openly about what receiving treatment and care felt like to them from the inside and which became a formative experience for Steven's students, helping them to recognise how easy it can be for well-meaning care to be felt as patronising often due to erroneous projections about mental health. In fact, these young people knew a great deal about their own difficulties and wanted to collaborate in their treatment rather that have interventions done to them. The opportunity to come into a university and speak as experts from experience was a profoundly empowering moment for them too. It is in this same spirit of generosity and collaboration that Walker's book is written. It offers much by way of up-to-date research and exploration of the central issues that any practitioner should be aware of, but it is a certain openness and acceptance of children and young people in all their social complexity and an example of a truly therapeutic approach that is this book's extra gift.

Chris Nicholson
Head of Department of Psychosocial and
Psychoanalytic Studies, University of Essex

BIBLIOGRAPHY

Wilson, P in Claveirole, A, Gaughan, M (eds) (2011) *Understanding Child and Young People's Mental Health* (p 15). London: Wiley-Blackwell.

Mind (2010) We need to talk: getting the right therapy at the right time. [online] Available at: www.mind.org.uk/media/280583/We-Need-to-Talk-getting-the-right-therapy-at-the-right-time.pdf (accessed 11 April 2019).

Timimi, S in House, R and Loewenthal, D (eds) (2009) *Childhood Wellbeing and a Therapeutic Ethos*. London: Karnac

Introduction

There can be no keener revelation of a society's soul than the way in which it treats its children.

Nelson Mandela

Evidence of the level of mental health problems in young people has been emerging for many years. The NSPCC reported that in 2018 the number of referrals by schools in England seeking mental health treatment for pupils has risen by more than a third over the last three years (The Guardian, 2018). The Nuffield Trust published research in September 2018 analysing mental health and well-being trends among children and young people over the past two decades (Pitchforth et al, 2018). They looked at data from 140,830 participants aged between 4 and 24 across 36 national surveys in England, Scotland and Wales. They found a striking, six-fold increase in how many children and young people in England reported having a long-standing mental health condition between 1995 and 2014 (from 0.8 to 4.8 per cent). And among young adults between 16 and 24, there was a ten-fold increase from 0.6 per cent to just under 6 per cent.

Increasing numbers of teenagers in England and Wales are killing themselves according to the UK Office for National Statistics (2017). The data shows that there were 177 suicides among 15 to 19 year olds in 2017, compared with 110 in 2010 and more than in every year since then except 2015, when the toll was 186. Fifty-six girls and women in the age group killed themselves last year, the highest number since records began in 1981. The suicide rate among that group, 3.5 per 100,000 people, was also the highest on record, and well up on the rate of 2.1 per 100,000 in 2010. The suicide rate among boys and men that age climbed to 7.1 per 100,000. There were 121 young male suicides in 2018 compared to 74 in 2010.

The number of girls under the age of 18 being treated in hospital in England after self-harming has nearly doubled compared with 20 years ago, according to NHS figures released in 2018 (Morgan et al, 2017). The figure reached 13,463 in 2018 against 7,327 in 1997. The number of girls treated for attempting a substance overdose has risen more than tenfold to 2,736 last year from 249 in 1997, while the number of boys treated increased over the past 21 years from 152 to 839 in 2017.

The Care Quality Commission (CQC) reported in late 2017 that child and adolescent mental health services (CAMHS) are overwhelmed with demand, and young people are waiting up to 18 months to be treated (Care Quality Commission, 2018). The CQC warned that long delays for treatment are damaging the health of young people with anxiety, depression and other conditions. In the same year, the Children's Commissioner

(2018) expressed her concerns that only between a quarter and a fifth of children with mental health conditions received help in 2018.

In 2017 the government published a Green Paper laying out their plans for children and young people's mental health services following criticism and pressure from parents, young people and professionals witnessing unprecedented increases in mental health problems among young people (DHSC, 2017). The proposals include introducing mental health support teams (linked to groups of schools and colleges), designated leads for mental health in all schools, new guidance for schools that will address the effect of trauma and a four-week waiting-time target across CAMHS.

This book has been written and designed in a way to enable any worker involved in supporting, helping and caring for young people to use it as a practical resource in their work as teachers, social workers, nurses, youth workers, doctors, foster carers, residential staff, psychologists and psychiatrists. Parents and young people will also find much of value in the book. I have tried to write in a jargon-free, accessible way with activities, questions, reflective commentary and case studies designed to relate to relatively common situations in this field of work. I hope this book provides you with the necessary inspiration, knowledge and skills to be able to engage more confidently in this area of work and, above all, enable you to reflect on your practice, your feelings about this topic and on your own history so that by combining these experiences, you can offer the most important resource to troubled young people – yourself.

Chapter 1 provides guidance on how to recognise emerging mental health problems and how these are defined and diagnosed in the professional literature.

The importance of the different perceptions of mental illness is explored together with a discussion about the vexed issue of the causes. There is information about the stages of children's developmental stages and how this interacts with concepts of personality development. Finally, there are tips on how to develop critical/reflective practice together with sociological perspectives on the challenges faced by young people today.

Chapter 2 outlines the principles underlying assessment in child and adolescent mental health with particular reference to useful resources that embrace a more holistic picture of the young person by assessing their strengths as well as the negative behaviour causing concern. The importance of being alert to the early warning signs of mental illness is emphasised, together with the role that stress can play in the propensity to develop problems. There is guidance on risk factors, the role of early child sexual abuse and important guidance on how to nurture resilience in young people.

Chapter 3 contains extensive evidence and supportive guidance on the particular mental health needs of socially excluded young people and those from black, Asian and minority ethnic backgrounds at risk of developing problems. The importance of ensuring that support services are accessible and culturally appropriate, and considerations of to what extent religion and spirituality are meaningful to young people are underlined. The needs of young people with learning disabilities, young offenders and those looked after are often neglected, so this chapter offers clear guidance and information to ensure they get proper attention and support.

Chapter 4 provides clear guidance on how to prepare support for the young person, and crucially what can be done to prevent mental health problems developing in the first place. Strategies for making sure your interventions are empowering for the young person are illustrated, with guidance on how to develop reflective practice and a range of skills to use in your support. The importance of integrated working is emphasised with tips on how to reduce the barriers between and within services. Mindfulness is becoming an increasingly important tool in this area of work so this appears in the form of simple, effective exercises to consider using in your work/home context.

Chapter 5 focuses on ways in which staff working with young people can help parents/carers better understand each other. There are explanations about teenage behaviour, developmental challenges and common issues that can make fraught situations worse in families. Alcohol and drugs are a big issue in the lives of young people and there is discussion about whether this is a cause or effect of mental health problems. Family-focused work is described as an intervention method to help improve communication and understanding between parents/carers and young people. The importance of harnessing the knowledge and wisdom of grandparents is emphasised, together with ways in which creative use of stories, legends and myths can be used to reach troubled children.

Chapter 6 examines the latest research and evidence base for determining what challenges young people are faced with in contemporary society. The new role envisaged for schools against the backdrop of budget cuts is discussed. The huge increase in self-harm among young women is considered with guidance on how to recognise this serious problem and provide appropriate, sensitive care and support. Attention deficit hyperactive disorder (ADHD) is considered in the context of prevalence and recent evidence on gender differences. The specific needs of traumatised refugee or asylum-seeking young people are outlined, and there are helpful guidance and suggestions for working with lesbian, gay, bisexual and transgender young people prone to developing mental health problems.

Chapter 7 concludes with a brief outline of the most up-to-date and important legislative and policy changes affecting young people's mental health in terms of their human rights. Specific guidance illustrates those areas of these various documents that can be accessed and integrated into your practice to ensure a children's rights perspective underpins all your work. In particular, the issues of confidentiality and consent to treatment are emphasised together with help on how to navigate the dilemmas often encountered. Finally, there is an opportunity for you to consider what your role is in this increasingly demanding and complex area which will manifest itself in any workplace where there are children and young people.

One of the most renowned and internationally acclaimed child psychiatrists Professor Michael Rutter wrote many years ago that children did not always need specialist support for their problems, instead suggesting that improvements in school, social and family situations offered a more effective outcome. He stressed that the greatest chance of positive change in children with conduct problems and emotional difficulties consistent with early signs of mental health problems lies mainly in improvements in their family circumstances, positive peer group relationships, good school experiences and less indirect contact with specialist child psychiatric services.

Terminology

The terms *children* and *young person* are used throughout this text generally to include people up to the age of 18 years. There are a wide variety of developmental and cognitive differences in young people; some young people have old heads on young shoulders while others are slow to mature. This means that generalising about a specific age group is problematic. The term *parent/carer* is used to highlight the important role played by non-biological adults in the upbringing of children and young people. *Family* is a term used in its broadest sense to incorporate diverse forms of social groupings that do not necessarily fit the nuclear, heterosexual majority model, such as same-sex couples, step-families and single-parent, foster and communal families. *Black* is used in the text to include every ethnic group subjected to institutional and personal racism that results in the devaluing of ethnic minority culture. The terms *psychological* or *mental health problems*, rather than disorder or illness, are used generically to cover psychiatric terminology that is not appropriate for the intended readership and to avoid unnecessary repetition of the variety and severity of different emotional and behavioural difficulties faced by children and young people. *Emotional well-being* is a term increasingly appearing in the modern literature and policy guidance regarding children and young people, and is used in this text synonymously with *mental health*. To avoid the use of gendered pronouns the singular *they* is used.

Chapter 1: What is mental illness and what is the extent of the problem?

Introduction

The spectrum of mental health problems covers a wide arc from 'normal', common, uncommon to complex and rare. This chapter will focus on how mental health problems are defined, how prevalent they are among young people, and will explore the link between child development and mental health problems commonly experienced by children and adolescents. The concept of 'normal' is highly problematic yet it is a term that regularly appears in textbooks and is used by professional staff to try to measure and quantify the individual experience of troubled young people.

Defining 'normal' is difficult due to the number of variables affecting a child or adolescent's behaviour or mood. Class, ethnicity, gender, language, culture, sexuality, religion and age are some of the factors that militate against generalising across populations. Within each factor there are sub-variables and distinctions, so for example it is problematic to make general assumptions about the age of adolescent transition and what is 'normal' behaviour at this time in a multicultural, ethnically rich and diverse society.

It is important to recognise that just because something is statistically common does not mean it is easier to manage; for an individual young person, their parents/carers, friends or teachers it can be part of complex and very difficult circumstances. It is not easy to distinguish between different levels of meaning and symptom severity as we shall see later on, but the available evidence will be evaluated to help you feel better able to understand what might be happening in certain situations you are likely to encounter and how you can use knowledge and skills to make a positive difference. The task is not helped by a variety of terms used by doctors, psychiatrists and psychologists in general or specialist contexts to describe often the same thing. Thus we find the terms *mental illness*, *mental health problem* and *mental disorder* used interchangeably. Their use with children and young people and/or their parents/carers is also problematic because of the impact such language might have and where other explanations for odd behaviour or changes in mood have previously been offered.

Workers themselves may be very hesitant to use essentially medical language and descriptions when assessing children and young people. The word *mental* can trigger a variety of associations and responses often conditioned by individual, family and societal attitudes. Media representations of mental illness can reinforce or sometimes challenge stereotypes. Plus, research demonstrates that there is still considerable stigma attached to the label *mental illness/disorder* or *problem* with children themselves reflecting adult prejudice, ignorance and rank fear (Walker, 2011a). Staff and parents are not immune to such beliefs and influences but it is important that you keep an open mind and do not quickly leap to wrongly diagnose or equally deny that a child may be developing mental health problems.

The task of gathering information about possible causative factors of child mental health problems is complicated by the fact that it is adult carers, worried about children, not the children themselves, that usually present asking for help. Children may not agree with parental interpretations of events and indeed may not even accept that there is a problem at all.

Prevalence and problems

Recent evidence indicates that 10 per cent of children up to the age of 18 years in Britain have a diagnosable mental health disorder (The Guardian, 2018). Higher rates exist among those living in inner city environments. One in five children and adolescents have a mental health problem which, although less serious, still requires professional support. Mental health problems include depression, anxiety, self-harm and disturbed behavior, and 70 per cent of children and young people who experience a mental health problem have not had any help. Behaviour resulting from mental illness can be misunderstood as 'naughty' or 'lazy'. It has been further estimated that child and adolescent mental health services are only reaching a minority of the population in their catchment areas requiring help (Children's Commissioner, 2018).

This indicates that a large number of children and young people are not receiving the necessary support and help to relieve their suffering. Research shows for example that one in 17 adolescents have harmed themselves – representing 200,000 11 to 15 year olds. At the other end of the age spectrum, there are increasing numbers of children under seven years of age being excluded from school due to uncontrollable behavioural problems. In any average primary school there will be 20 children with mental health problems. In an average comprehensive/technical college there will be 100 students with mental health problems (Rodway et al, 2016).

The number of girls self-harming between the ages of 13 and 17 has risen by 70 per cent from 2014 to 2017 (Morgan et al, 2017). Data from the Office for National Statistics (2017) shows that in 2015 there were 168 males aged 10 to 19 and 63 females in the same age group who took their own lives. The total figure of 231 is the highest it has been since 2001 when 240 youngsters committed suicide. The increased rate of suicide over the last 28 years in children and adolescents is a cause of increasing concern and a stark indicator of the mental health of young people. The Children's Commissioner said that only between a quarter and a fifth of children with mental health conditions received help in 2016 and it bears repeating the revelation from the Care Quality Commission in 2017 that there was an 18-month waiting time for access to treatment (Care Quality Commission, 2018). In 2017, the President of the Family Division of the High Court condemned the *'disgraceful and utterly shaming lack of proper provision in this country'* for young people struggling with mental illness (The Guardian, 2017a).

Common mental health problems in young people

Depression

Depression is one of the most common child and adolescent mental health problems. In order to understand the nature of the low mood a child or adolescent may be experiencing, the following guidance can help in measuring in some way the intensity of the depression and help you organise an appropriate response. An initial assessment should ascertain whether at least one of the following symptoms is present on most days, most of the time or for at least the last two weeks: persistent sadness or low (irritable) mood, loss of interests and/or pleasure and fatigue or low energy. If any of these are present, you should find out about associated symptoms that may be experienced, such as those below. Then ask about any past history of depression, family history, associated disability and availability of social support.

- Poor or increased sleep.

- Poor concentration or indecisiveness.

- Low self-confidence.

- Poor or increased appetite.

- Suicidal thoughts or acts.

- Agitation or slowing of movements.

- Guilt or self-blame.

If the young person has four or fewer of the above symptoms, has no past or family history of depression and has some social support available, then it may not be serious. If these symptoms are intermittent, or of less than two weeks in duration, the young person is not actively suicidal and has little associated disability, then your intervention can rely on providing general advice and 'watchful waiting'.

If the young person has five or more of the above symptoms together with a past history or family history of depression and a low level of social support, then the depression is more serious. Combined with suicidal thoughts and associated social disability, more active help will be required in primary care and the GP should be contacted to arrange an appointment. Together with the GP, you may decide after the first appointment that a referral to a mental health professional at Tier 2 CAMHS is necessary if the young person is not coping, neglecting themselves, their relatives are more concerned or there is a recurrent episode of depression within one year of the first. If the following factors are present then an urgent referral to a child psychiatrist is needed.

- Active suicidal ideas or plans.

- Psychotic symptoms.

- Severe agitation accompanying severe (seven or more) symptoms.

- Severe self-neglect.

Suicide

Suicide warrants particular attention for obvious reasons. It is worth considering the commonly accepted definition as well as other related terms such as *parasuicide* and *deliberate self-harm* to appreciate the differences between these terms and how they can get confused. Suicide refers to death that directly or indirectly results from an act that the dead person believed would result in this end. The definition of deliberate self-harm includes non-fatal or attempted suicide, but also life-threatening behaviours such as self-poisoning in which the young person does not intend to take their life as well as habitual cutting, piercing and head banging. Parasuicide is defined as serious but unsuccessful attempts to kill oneself such as any deliberate act with a non-fatal outcome that appears to cause or actually causes self-harm, or would have done so without intervention from others.

Recent evidence confirms for example that suicide is of particular concern in marginalised and victimised adolescent groups including gay, lesbian and bisexual youth. Research such as that by Bhui and McKenzie (2008) suggests that despite the rhetoric of anti-discriminatory policies and professional statements of equality, heterosexist and homophobic attitudes continue to be displayed by some psychologists and social workers. This can further reinforce feelings of rejection, confusion and despair in troubled young people. Other evidence warns against a narrow definition of sexual-minority adolescents that pathologises their behaviour or wrongly assumes a higher risk of self-harming behaviour (Walker, 2016).

Adolescents at risk of suicide can feel that they can resolve their internal states of despair and angst by splitting away from their body. Thus, by killing their physical body, they believe they can liberate their psychic self from the emotional pain and suffering. Adolescents at risk of psychosis are often suicidal, but suicide is not the outcome in many cases. Working with adolescents who are suicidal means being exposed to intense and extreme emotions such as anxiety, guilt, responsibility and fear. It is highly problematic to work with because it is immune to predictability and because there are multiple aspects to suicidality.

Anxiety

Fears and anxieties are normal developmental challenges facing the maturing young person. The relative intensity, frequency and duration of the behaviour associated with anxiety needs to be evaluated, and their role in the course of normal development considered against the frequency of the same behaviours among non-troubled children from the same class, culture and ethnic background. There are three main anxiety problems experienced by children and adolescents:

Generalised anxiety disorder

This is usually characterised by unrealistic and excessive anxiety and worry that do not seem to be linked to a specific situation or external stress. Children like this tend to worry about future events such as family activities, health issues and exams or just what is going to happen in the next hour or day. A young person in a chronic state of being on edge constantly can be understood as being in a state of anxious apprehension.

Obsessive compulsive disorder

This involves recurrent obsessions or compulsions that are time-consuming, cause distress and lead to problems in everyday functioning. Intrusive thoughts or images are also characteristic and perceived as senseless and inappropriate. Common themes are contamination, dirt, violence, harm or religious concepts. Washing rituals are particularly common.

Separation anxiety disorder

This is related to children usually and focuses on distress caused from and about being separated from those with whom the child is attached. It usually features children refusing to sleep away from home, staying excessively close to a parent at home, and particularly problems around the time of starting school. Children are often fearful of some unspecific harm befalling their important attachment figures. School phobia is a variation of this problem and occurs when an anxious child can be comfortable in any setting other than school.

Autism

Autism has probably been around for a lot longer than the first recorded diagnosis and definition in the early 1940s. Like many problems before and since, it can be evidenced in children and young people in hindsight but until the 1940s there were different explanations for those showing the characteristics we nowadays associate with autism. The cause of the problem is still the subject of constant research and much controversy (Doherty et al, 2016) but there are associations with physical disorders (ie rubella) suggesting organic pathology as one important factor. A brief definition of autism is: *'abnormal development of language and social relationships with ritualistic and obsessional behaviours'* (Walker, 2011a, p 76). Key characteristics of a child or young person with autism are:

• failure to comprehend others' feelings, lack of interest in imitative or social play, and inability to seek friendships or comfort from others;

• impairments in verbal and non-verbal communication and avoidance of eye contact;

• resistance to change and limited interests.

Assessing autism accurately is notoriously difficult, especially in pre-school-age children when normal lack of socialisation and ranges in verbal communication vary widely. It is only when children attend school that those with autism tend to be identified because of the different way they behave and relate to others. It is also difficult to be certain about the prevalence of autism in the population. This is due to the complex classification systems used by health and psychiatric professionals and the way contemporary research has identified a variety of different conditions along the autistic spectrum of behaviour (Doherty et al, 2016). What is certain is that as diagnosis and assessment skills improve in health and social care staff, more children and young people are being identified and diagnosed with autism. Current estimates suggest a prevalence rate in the general population of between 7 and 17 per 10,000 children (National Austistic Society, nd).

Autism begins at birth but tends to be unrecognised until the child is two to three years old. There is usually a delay between parent concerns and diagnosis. This can be explained by the general lack of knowledge around child development but especially among primary health care staff who are untrained or cautious about offering an opinion. By the age of three however, both parents and health care staff usually concur that autism could be the cause of the language delay and lack of peer relationships. In addition, other people such as friends, neighbours or nursery staff are reporting the pronounced lack of sociability, inability to empathise or capacity to reflect on social situations. This then quickly leads to social isolation in play groups or nurseries, reinforcing the characteristic preference of an autistic child for solitary repetitive play.

Autism is found 75 per cent more often in boys than girls and half of all autistic individuals never speak (National Autistic Society, nd). Those that can show unusual use of language in their intonation, stress placed on various words and often speak in a monotone. A significant proportion of autistic children have behavioural and emotional problems expressed in hyperactivity, short attention span, aggression, self-harm and anxiety/depression. Autistic features are often present where there is a generalised learning disability.

Repetitive behaviour is a major symptom of autism but there are a variety of motivations that contribute to the behaviour's occurrence – anxiety, self-soothing, self-stimulation and some more desultory states where the child may be deeply bored but not know it; or, may not know how to seek out and shift to another more interesting activity. Where the activity has built up to a frenzy, the child may need to be distracted with a fairly exciting alternative. The importance of enlisting parents as co-therapists in behavioural treatments is crucial. Helping them learn problem-solving skills is important in their ongoing management of current and future behavioural problems.

Asperger's syndrome

A precise diagnosis and definition is difficult to obtain because there is still confusion between autism and Asperger's in medical and health literature. A child with Asperger's is likely to have better cognitive and communication skills but still experience poor social interaction and stereotyped interests. It is estimated that the prevalence rates for Asperger's are higher than for autism but there is little robust evidence in this area. This is partly explained by the relatively high levels of intelligence found in such children, which can serve to mask other difficulties especially during adolescence. Asperger's is more prevalent in boys and can be characterised by a notable physical clumsiness with a very characteristic monotonous speech pattern and inflection. Anxiety, depression and low self-esteem are particularly found in adolescence. As yet, there is no definitive treatment or support but your role would include:

• assessment needs to highlight the strengths of the child;

- parent education and support to help them understand and cope;

- early identification required to intervene with social and language skills.

Drug, alcohol and substance misuse

Young people in the UK are more likely to drink alcohol excessively and get involved in drug use much more than their counterparts in mainland Europe. Workers should consider whether the drug and alcohol misuse is a cause of mental health problems or a consequence. Alcohol and drug abuse are factors associated with anti-social behaviour, criminal activity and poor educational attainment. The interim period between adolescence and adulthood is the highest-risk period for problematic drug use. This is especially so for those individuals described as externalised (the under-parented) and the internalised (the over-parented).

These young people grow up in family units of two extremes. The externalised family tend to be permissive and exert little control over the development of the young person, model poor behaviour around high consumption and exert little influence on the peer groups that their children subscribe too. The internalised group tend to be abstinent, fretful parents who over-protect their offspring from risk and responsibility, censure peer contact and thus disconnect their children from the socialisation process.

Self-harm

Self-harm among young people is a major public health issue in the UK. It affects at least one in 15 young people and some evidence suggests that rates of self-harm in the UK are higher than anywhere else in Europe (Walker, 2012a). Self-harm blights the lives of young people and seriously affects their relationships with families and friends. It presents a major challenge to all those in services and organisations that work with young people, from schools through to hospital accident and emergency departments. Levels of self-harm are one indicator of the mental health and mental well-being of young people in our society in general. Due to the increased prevalence data emerging from the latest research, refer to Chapter 6 for more guidance on this particular problem.

Eating disorders

Assessment of young people with eating disorders should be comprehensive and include physical, psychological and social needs, and a comprehensive assessment of risk to self. The level of risk to the young person's mental and physical health should be monitored as treatment progresses because it may increase – for example, following weight change or at times of transition between services in cases of anorexia nervosa

(NICE, 2017). For people with eating disorders presenting in primary care, GPs should take responsibility for the initial assessment and the initial co-ordination of care. This includes the determination of the need for emergency medical or mental health assessment.

Young people and, where appropriate, carers, should be provided with education and information on the nature, course and treatment of eating disorders. In addition to the provision of information, family and carers may be informed of self-help groups and support groups, and offered the opportunity to participate in such groups where they exist. Staff should acknowledge that many people with eating disorders are ambivalent about treatment and recognise the consequent demands and challenges this presents. Young people with eating disorders should be assessed and receive treatment at the earliest opportunity. Early treatment is particularly important for those with or at risk of severe emaciation and they should be prioritised for treatment.

Anorexia nervosa

Most people with anorexia nervosa should be managed in the community with psychological treatment provided by a service that is competent in giving that treatment and assessing the physical risk of people with eating disorders. Young people with anorexia nervosa requiring in-patient treatment should be admitted to a setting that can provide the skilled implementation of re-feeding with careful physical monitoring (particularly in the first few days of re-feeding) in combination with psycho-social interventions. Family interventions that directly address the eating disorder should be offered to children and adolescents with anorexia nervosa.

Feeding against the will of the patient

Feeding against the will of the patient should be an intervention of the last resort, and only undertaken in the care and management of anorexia nervosa. Feeding against the will of the patient is a highly specialised procedure requiring expertise in the care and management of those with severe eating disorders and the physical complications associated with them. This should only be done in the context of the Mental Health Act 1983 or Children Act 1989. When making the decision to feed against the will of the patient, the legal basis for any such action must be clear.

Bulimia nervosa

As a possible first step, young people with bulimia nervosa should be encouraged to follow an evidence-based self-help programme. The course of treatment should be for 16 to 20 sessions over four to five months. Adolescents with bulimia nervosa may be treated with CBT-BN, adapted as needed to suit their age, circumstances and level of development, and including the family as appropriate.

For all eating disorders

Family members, including siblings, should normally be included in the treatment of children and adolescents with eating disorders. Interventions may include sharing of information, advice on behavioural management, and facilitating communication. In children and adolescents with eating disorders, growth and development should be closely monitored. Where development is delayed or growth is stunted despite adequate nutrition, paediatric advice should be sought. Staff assessing children and adolescents with eating disorders should be alert to indicators of abuse (emotional, physical and sexual) and should remain so throughout treatment.

The right to confidentiality of children and adolescents with eating disorders should be respected. When working with children and adolescents with eating disorders, workers should familiarise themselves with national guidelines and their employers' policies in the area of confidentiality. In the absence of evidence to guide the management of atypical eating disorders (eating disorders not otherwise specified) other than binge eating disorder, it is recommended to follow the guidance on the treatment of the eating problem that most closely resembles the individual patient's eating disorder.

Schizophrenia

This is best understood as a collection of several disorders rather than one single mental health problem. It is nothing to do with 'split personality'. It is uncommon in early adolescence but prevalence increases with age and in males. The signs to watch out for are:

- psychotic state with delusions, hallucinations or thought disorders;

- significant reduction in social contact;

- deterioration in general and academic functioning;

- reduction in personal care and hygiene;

- lack of emotional affect in some young people;

- lack of energy or spontaneity;

- lack of enjoyment.

Risk factors include:

- family history;

- biochemical and brain disorder;

- substance misuse which triggers psychosis.

The treatment and management of schizophrenia has been divided into three phases: initiation of treatment at the first episode; acute phase; and promoting recovery. As a worker you might be involved at any or all of these phases.

The national guidelines make good practice points and recommendations for psychological, pharmacological and service-level interventions in the three phases of care in both primary care and secondary mental health services.

The effects of schizophrenia on a young person's life experience and opportunities are considerable. Service users and carers need help and support to deal with their future and to cope with the changes the illness brings. Workers should work in partnership with service users and carers, offering help, treatment and care in an atmosphere of hope and optimism. For most young people experiencing a schizophrenic breakdown, the level of distress, anxiety and subjective confusion, especially during first episodes, leads to difficulty in accessing services. Service users and their relatives seeking help should be assessed and receive treatment at the earliest possible opportunity

The focus of your intervention and joint work is to help improve the experience and outcomes of care for people with schizophrenia. These outcomes include:

- the degree of symptomatic recovery;

- quality of life;

- degree of personal autonomy;

- ability and access to work;

- stability and quality of living accommodation;

- degree and quality of social integration;

- degree of financial independence;

- the experience and impact of side effects.

The assessment of health and social care needs for young people with schizophrenia should therefore be comprehensive, and address medical, social, psychological, educational, economic, physical and cultural issues.

Attention deficit hyperactivity disorder (ADHD)

ADHD is for some staff and health professionals a controversial subject where it is believed by some that there is over-diagnosis and over-use of stimulant medication to control children's natural boisterous behaviour, or that the problem of ADHD is more widespread and under-diagnosed. Diagnosis of ADHD has multiplied in recent years as have concerns about the short- and long-term side effects of drug treatment. Others accept that it is a real problem and a behavioural syndrome characterised by the core symptoms of hyperactivity, impulsivity and inattention. While these symptoms tend to cluster together, some children are predominantly hyperactive and impulsive, while others are principally inattentive. Not every young person with ADHD has all of the symptoms of hyperactivity, impulsivity and inattention. However, for a person to be diagnosed with ADHD, their symptoms should be associated with at least a moderate degree of psychological, social and/or educational impairment.

Moderate ADHD in children and young people is present when the symptoms of hyperactivity, impulsivity and/or inattention, or all three, occur together, and are associated with at least moderate impairment, which should be present in multiple settings (for example, home and school or a health care setting) and in multiple domains such as achievement in schoolwork or homework; dealing with physical risks and avoiding common hazards; and forming positive relationships with family and peers, where the level appropriate to the child's chronological and mental age has not been reached. Determining the severity of the disorder should be a matter for clinical judgement, taking into account the severity of impairment, pervasiveness, individual factors and familial and social context.

What are the causes of child and adolescent mental health problems?

Research into the causes of problems (Walker, 2011a) reveals very complex, often interrelated, causal factors in relation to young people's mental health. Two aspects of causation should not be confused:

- **Individual differences:** in the liability to develop difficulties, in the course of those difficulties and in the extent to which they recur.

- **Group differences:** for example, between the sexes (asking why a certain increase is greater among boys or girls) or between different ethnic groups.

It is important to look at the influence of the context and environment on an individual, at why a susceptibility to difficulty actually translates into, for example, a mental health problem or anti-social act. Risk factors are typically considered but are not always indicative so a young person with high numbers of risk factors may not develop mental health problems, whereas someone with low numbers does. The death of a parent or loss due to divorce/separation is associated with depression, but it is the *impaired parenting* that follows the loss that triggers the depression, not the loss itself.

Why has there been an increase in mental health problems among young people?

The UK has seen an increase in family disruption, in educational expectations and demand for scholastic credentials, in major decision-making (regarding for example drugs and sex) and in prolongation of financial dependence on parents. Environmental factors could include greater cultural conflict, media images at odds with reality, toxins and pollutants, greater inequality and a decline in social cohesion and responsibility.

Here is a list of factors to bear in mind when trying to understand why a young person may be becoming mentally ill.

- Family dysfunction: separation, divorce.

- Racism, homophobia.

- Sexual, physical or psychological abuse.

- Economic stress: unemployment, poor housing, low income, poverty, debt.

- School stress: exam pressure, bullying, league tables, budget cuts, low staff morale.

- Access to drugs or alcohol.

- Cyberbullying, internet culture, violent video games, pornography.

- Genetic factors; biological and neurological issues.

- Parental mental illness.

- The pace of modern life.

It is useful to the discussion about definitions and distinctions to make a distinction between mental health problems and mental health disorders. Problems are defined as a disturbance of function in one area of relationships, mood or behaviour, or development of sufficient severity to require professional intervention. Mental health disorders are defined as either a severe problem, commonly persistent, or the co-occurrence of a number of problems, usually in the presence of a number of risk factors. This can be translated into some descriptions of the more common disorders of mental health found in children and adolescents.

- Emotional disorders (phobias, anxiety states, depression).

- Conduct disorders (stealing, defiance, fire-setting, aggression, anti-social behaviour).

- Hyperkinetic disorders (disturbance of activity and attention, ADHD).

- Developmental disorders (autism, speech delay, poor bladder control).

- Eating disorders (infant eating problems, anorexia nervosa, bulimia).

- Habit disorders (tics, sleeping problems, soiling).

- Somatic disorders (chronic fatigue syndrome).

- Psychotic disorders (schizophrenia, manic depression, drug-induced psychoses).

Schizophrenia represents one of the most serious, rare and controversial disorders classified by psychiatrists. Until relatively recently, child and adolescent psychiatrists had previously considered that the onset of schizophrenia only occurred in late adolescence. However, there is growing evidence that younger children are experiencing this most severe form of mental health problems without receiving adequate help and support. Part of the reason for this is the general reluctance to diagnose such a disorder because of fears about the potentially adverse consequences of the label, but there is also a history of uncertainty and lack of reliable classification instruments with which to apply a core definition across the variety of childhood developmental stages.

Table 1.1 Problem, disorder or illness?

Mental health problem	Common difficulties recognised as typically of brief duration and not requiring any formal professional intervention.
Mental health disorder	Abnormalities of emotions, behaviour or social relationships sufficiently marked or prolonged to cause suffering or risk to optimal development in the child, or distress or disturbance in the child or community.
Mental illness	A clinically recognisable set of symptoms or behaviour associated in most cases with considerable distress and substantial interference with personal functions.

Definitions and distinctions

The terms *mental health problem*, *mental health disorder* and *mental illness* are often used synonymously in both professional practice contexts and in the evidence-based literature. This can be confusing, particularly for non-specialists and service users and their families. Table 1.1 offers a guide to help clarify the differences between these terms and how to measure their use in particular situations.

Mental health problems can be distinguished by the term *disorder*, by the degree of seriousness and the length of time the condition lasts. The assumption is that most people will recognise these symptoms and understand they do not require specialist or intensive intervention. Note the idea of abnormality of emotions and the notion of them being sufficiently marked or prolonged. This parallel is useful in as much as it reveals how imprecise these definitions are and how open they are to interpretation. Who decides what is abnormal: the worker, parent or child? How is the notion of sufficiently marked or prolonged measured and against what standard? Mental illness takes us into the realm of medicine and the clinical guidelines and diagnostic criteria usually applied to the most serious difficulties and those that are statistically rare. At the other end of the scale, the terms *emotional well-being* or *emotional literacy* are becoming popular among the wider public and professionals even though it would be hard to find agreement about a definition of what these terms mean.

Different perceptions

The behaviour and emotional affect of children and young people diagnosed with symptoms of mental health difficulty can be considered in different ways within a variety of professional and public discourses. The dominant discourse is that of medicine and especially psychiatry, which continues to refine classifications of symptoms into universal descriptors. Yet behaviour and expressed emotions can be interpreted widely, depending on the theoretical base of the professional involved and the specific cultural and historical context of their manifestation.

The term *mental illness* was constructed in the context of a debate among psychiatrists about the criteria for diagnosing specific mental health problems. Previously they had relied on a constellation of symptoms based on adult measures to distinguish children and adolescents whose condition was outside the normal experience. There are limitations in psychiatric diagnosis and by implication, the medical model it embodies. Not all children with symptoms of mental disorder show marked impairment, and conversely, some children have significant psycho-social impairment without reaching the clinical threshold for diagnosis.

If it is problematic to define mental *illness* or disorder, then it is equally difficult to define what is meant by mental *health* for children and young people. It can mean different things to families, children or professionals, and staff from different professional backgrounds might not share the same perception of what mental health is. A common set of characteristics that show mental health in childhood and adolescence is present includes:

• a capacity to enter into and sustain mutually satisfying personal relationships;

• a continuing progression of psychological development;

• an ability to play and to learn so that attainments are appropriate for age and intellectual level;

• a developing moral sense of right and wrong;

• the degree of psychological distress and maladaptive behaviour being within normal limits for the child's age and context.

Defined in this way, mental health is a rather ideal state, which depends upon the potential and experience of each individual, and is maintained or hindered by external circumstances and events. The Mental Health Foundation suggests that children who are mentally healthy will have the ability to:

• **develop** psychologically, emotionally, creatively, intellectually and physically;

• **initiate**, develop and sustain mutually satisfying personal relationships;

- **use** and enjoy solitude;

- **become** aware of others and empathise with them;

- **play** and learn;

- **develop** a sense of right and wrong;

- **resolve** (face) problems and setbacks and learn from them.

The World Health Organization (2005) defines good mental health among children and adolescents as:

Able to achieve and maintain optimal psychological and social functioning and well-being. They have a sense of identity and self-worth, sound family and peer relationships, an ability to be productive and to learn, and a capacity to tackle developmental challenges and use cultural resources to maximise growth.

Workers practising in a holistic context will be attuned to the social dimension affecting children's mental health. They need to consider how they define the terms *mental disorder* and *mental health* and whether their practice aims to help children and young people 'adjust to the stress of everyday living' or challenge those stresses within a personal helping relationship.

These definitions and the subtle distinctions between mental illness and mental health are important in the sense that they set the context for how parents and professionals and others conceptualise difficulties experienced by children and young people. Examples later on in this text will illustrate how education, youth justice and social work staff can all offer quite different explanations for the same behaviour with significantly different outcomes to intervention. So it is very important to be as clear as you can be about what it is you are observing and what sources of knowledge are informing those perceptions. Acquiring a label of mental illness can not only be stigmatising in the short term but can have profound longer-term consequences for a young person in terms of relationships, employment, education and personal health or life insurance.

✒ Activity 1.1 Case illustration

You are a teacher in a primary school and responsible for a class of 10 year olds. One child is persistently loud, interrupts you and is affecting other children. The child does not seem able to concentrate, and normal interventions to stop the behaviour are failing.

Chapter 1: What is mental illness and what is the extent of the problem?

21

The child is a black boy from a single parent family living in poor housing conditions. You feel angry with this boy because he is distracting you and other children. He is removed from the class. In discussions with your head of year and the boy's parent you discover that his father recently died in a prolonged period of critical illness.

⬭ Commentary

With more information you have been able to place the child's behaviour in a wider context. The impact on this child and the rest of the family of the father's terminal illness and subsequent death has been disturbing and distressing, resulting in anxiety which prevents concentration and learning and is expressed in distracting behaviour within class. With new information, your feelings of irritation and anger have shifted to those of care, concern and guilt. Now you can work together with pastoral care, his mother and other colleagues to try to mitigate his impact on others, get him support to modify his behaviour and monitor him to see whether his behaviour becomes worse and more disturbed, requiring referral to or consultation by CAMHS.

Recognition

Growing evidence for the difference in professional perceptions of mental health problems in young people is shown by a recent survey conducted among GPs (O'Brien et al, 2017). It revealed that they were only identifying 10 per cent of children attending GP surgeries who had some form of severe psychological or emotional problem. These findings are worrying because primary care is one of the most crucial gateways for children and young people to gain access to appropriate services and resources and for signposting to accessible and acceptable support in this area. Different professionals and parents will view a child's behaviour through a different lens resulting in a diversity of opinions and assumptions about what is wrong. This reflects the value and knowledge base of each person coming into contact with a child, influenced by cultural norms, stereotypes and expectations. For example, a teenager with a history of anti-social behaviour may be perceived by youth justice staff as displaying criminal tendencies, whereas a social worker may view the same child as suffering from neglect, social exclusion and inconsistent parenting. A CAMHS worker may diagnose underlying untreated depression at the root of the problem behaviour.

Up until relatively recently, the different theoretical approaches to understanding the origin of children's mental health problems existed in isolation from each other. When brought together they were more likely to lead to competitive discussion and rivalry than thoughtful reflection and critical analysis. The polarised nature versus nurture debate is largely in the past and the interrelationships between the factors associated with child developmental outcomes are now widely acknowledged to be complex. We have moved far away from assuming that factors associated with risk are necessarily the direct cause of problems. Likewise, we no longer consider risk factors alone without also taking into account factors that promote resilience in children and young people. Simplistic statements that promote single causes of mental health problems in children, whether it be the role of diet, poverty, genes or other relevant associated factors, are misleading.

Is there a consensus emerging on the causes of CAMH problems?

• Individual differences are important: people react differently to similar stimuli that can be social, biochemical or environmental. Some of these individual differences may be genetically influenced.

• Nature versus nurture is a false dichotomy – too many factors intervene to alter possible or probable causal pathways. Our genes merely determine predispositions, not precise outcomes.

• We need to take far more seriously the associative connections that undoubtedly exist between mind and body, which seem to be stronger than many suppose.

• What children eat (nutrition) and young people's perceptions of and reactions to stress (cortisol and its aftermath) undoubtedly affect the biochemistry of their brains and bodies in fundamental ways. This is likely to affect behaviour patterns and control mechanisms (impulsivity).

• When identifying solutions, it is vital to differentiate between the predicament/ environment of a particular individual and that of the group (age, area, socio-economic status, ethnicity).

• The origins of mental health issues in adults will invariably lie in past experiences.

• Socio-economic status can have a profound impact on individual behaviour, for a range of different reasons, and these must be assessed carefully.

• Mental health problems and disorders can be viewed as the outcome of impaired, delayed or otherwise inhibited normal healthy development; as a rational yet often dysfunctional reaction to a difficult or challenging context; and as a dysfunctional, more extreme manifestation of an otherwise normal and functional state of mind.

Child and adolescent development

Understanding the key elements of human growth and developing theoretical resources relevant to young people's mental health are critical when seeking to understand and then plan to assess and intervene appropriately in the lives of troubled young people. Summaries have been provided below. They have been simplified to aid clarity and comparison and should be seen as part of a wide spectrum of potential, rather than deterministic, interactive causative factors in the genesis of child and adolescent mental health problems. Some social psychologists criticise the emphasis in child development theories on normative concepts and suggest enhancing the judging, measuring approach towards one that embodies context, culture and competencies. The following summaries should be adapted to every individual situation encountered and always considered against the white, Eurocentric perceptions they embodied when first constructed.

Freud's psychosexual stages of development

Year 1: The oral stage during which the infant obtains its principle source of comfort from sucking the breast milk of the mother, and the gratification from the nutrition.

Years 2–3: The anal stage when the anus and defecation are the major sources of sensual pleasure. The child is preoccupied with body control with parental/carer encouragement. Obsessional behaviour and over-control later in childhood could indicate a problematic stage of development.

Years 4–5: The phallic stage, with the vagina and penis the focus of attention, is the characteristic of this psychosexual stage. In boys the Oedipus complex and in girls the Electra complex are generated in desires to have a sexual relationship with the opposite-sex parent. The root of anxieties and neuroses can be found here if transition to the next stage is impeded.

Years 6–11: The latency stage, which is characterised by calm after the storm of the powerful emotions preceding it.

Years 12–18: The genital stage whereby the individual becomes interested in opposite-sex partners as a substitute for the opposite-sex parent, and as a way of resolving the tensions inherent in Oedipal and Electra complexes.

Bowlby's attachment theory

The following scheme represents the process of healthy attachment formation. Mental health problems may develop if an interruption occurs in this process, if care is inconsistent, or if there is prolonged separation from the child's main carer.

Months 0–2: This stage is characterised by pre-attachment undiscriminating social responsiveness. The baby is interested in voices and faces and enjoys social interaction.

Months 3–6: The infant begins to develop discriminating social responses and experiments with attachments to different people. Familiar people elicit more response than strangers.

Months 7–36: Attachment to the main carer is prominent with the child showing separation anxiety when the carer is absent. The child actively initiates responses from the carer.

Years 3–18: The main carer's absences become longer, but the child develops a reciprocal attachment relationship. The child and developing young person begins to understand the carer's needs from a secure emotional base.

Erikson's psycho-social stages of development

Five of Eriksen's eight stages of development will be considered.

Year 1: The infant requires consistent and stable care in order to develop feelings of security. He/she begins to trust the environment but can also develop suspicion and insecurity. Deprivation at this stage can lead to emotional detachment throughout life and difficulties forming relationships.

Years 2–3: The child begins to explore and seeks some independence from parents/carers. A sense of autonomy develops but improved self-esteem can combine with feelings of shame and self-doubt. Failure to integrate this stage may lead to difficulties in social integration.

Years 4–5: The child needs to explore the wider environment and plan new activities. Begins to initiate activities but fears punishment and guilt as a consequence. Successful integration results in a confident person, but problems can produce deep insecurities.

Years 6–11: The older child begins to acquire knowledge and skills to adapt to their surroundings. Develops a sense of achievement but marred by possible feelings of inferiority and failure if efforts are denigrated.

Years 12–18: The individual enters the stage of personal and vocational identity formation. Self-perception heightened, but there is potential for conflict, confusion and strong emotions.

Paget's stages of cognitive development

Years 0–1.5: The sensory-motor stage is characterised by infants exploring their physicality and modifying their reflexes until they can experiment with objects and build a mental picture of things around them.

Years 1.5–7: The pre-operational stage when the child acquires language, makes pictures and participates in imaginative play. The child tends to be self-centred and fixed in their thinking, believing they are responsible for external events.

Years 7–12: The concrete operations stage when a child can understand and apply more abstract tasks such as sorting or measuring. This stage is characterised by less egocentric thinking and more relational thinking – differentiation between things. The complexity of the external world is beginning to be appreciated.

Years 12–18: The stage of formal operations characterised by the use of rules and problem-solving skills. The child moves into adolescence with increasing capacity to think abstractly and reflect on tasks in a deductive, logical way.

Personality development

A more recent view of personality development lists five factors that combine elements of the older more classic ways of understanding a child or adolescent together with notions of peer acceptability and adult perceptions.

• **Extroversion:** includes traits such as extroverted/introverted, talkative/quiet, bold/timid.

• **Agreeableness:** based on characteristics such as agreeable/disagreeable, kind/unkind, selfish/unselfish.

- **Conscientiousness:** reflects traits such as organised/disorganised, hardworking/lazy, reliable/unreliable, thorough/careless, practical/impractical.

- **Neuroticism:** based on traits such as stable/unstable, calm/angry, relaxed/tense, unemotional/emotional.

- **Openness to experience:** includes the concept of intelligence, together with level of sophistication, creativity, curiosity and cognitive style in problem-solving situations.

Sociological perspectives

In addition to the classic means of understanding child and adolescent development outlined above, there are other, less prominent but as important resources for workers to draw upon to help inform practice in this area. Sociology may be suffering from less emphasis in government policy and occupational standards guidance but it still offers a valuable conceptual tool to enable a rounded, holistic process of assessment and intervention with troubled children. Sociological explanations for child and adolescent mental health problems can be located in a macro understanding of the way childhood itself is considered and constructed by adults.

- Childhood is a social construction. It is neither a natural nor a universal feature of human groups but appears as a specific structural and cultural component of many societies.

- Childhood is a variable of social analysis. Comparative and cross-cultural analysis reveals a variety of childhoods rather than a single or universal phenomenon.

- Children's social relationships and cultures require study in their own right, independent of the perspective and concern of adults.

- Children are and must be seen as active in the construction and determination of their own lives, the lives of those around them and of the societies in which they live.

An examination of the experience of childhood around the world today shows how greatly varied it is, and how it has changed throughout history. Contemporary children in some countries are working from the ages of eight and independent from the age of 14, whereas in other countries some do not leave home or begin work until they are 21. The developmental norms above show how adults construct childhood and therefore how to measure children's progress and detect mental health problems. They are however set down as solid absolutes and are based on notions of adults' fears

Chapter 1: What is mental illness and what is the extent of the problem?

27

about risk and lack of confidence in children, and are rooted in adults' own childhood experiences. These theories have had positive effects but they have also restricted the field of vision required to fully engage with and understand children and adolescents.

✎ Activity 1.2

🔸 Together with a friend or colleague, each write down three lists of your own characteristics at age 14 as you felt them, as your parents saw you, and as your class teacher perceived you.

🔸 Note the similarities and differences, and think about and discuss together what concepts informed those differences.

💬 Commentary

Early childhood studies are beginning to challenge the orthodoxy in child development theories so that children are seen as accomplishing, living, competent persons rather than not yet quite fully formed people who are learning to become adults. The idea that the stages have to be accomplished sequentially ignores the different pace at which different children change according to external and other influences. Adults simply need to reflect on themselves to see that adults of the same developmental age can be at very different stages of emotional maturity, skill and capacity. Workers therefore need to use concepts of development and definitions of child and adolescent mental health problems cautiously and sceptically. An appreciation of how these concepts are constructed reflecting historical and cultural dominant values, and how they reinforce the power relationships between adults and children, is required. The central processes apart from physical changes are the critical process of development of self, the search for identity and the development of relationships and the changing nature of relationships.

How can critical/reflective practice be developed?

Supervision or professional consultation in the area of child and adolescent mental health is a crucial component of reflective practice. A manager with the skills to offer case consultation combined with management supervision is ideal but probably a rarity. Workers involved with families or in situations where child mental health problems are an issue require quality consultation separate from the administrative and managerial aspects of their work. A senior colleague or other professional might be the best resource as long as they can help the worker disentangle their own feelings from those being generated during intense work. Simple concepts such as transference and projection used in a pragmatic way can go a long way towards increasing effectiveness and clarity in confusing and worrying situations.

A child's behaviour could be assessed as genetic predisposition by a physician, a specific disease requiring treatment by a psychiatrist, cognitive distortions by a psychologist, repressed unconscious desires by a child psychotherapist, or a consequence of environmental disadvantage by a social worker. It is therefore important to acquire knowledge and understanding of these potentially competing narrative understandings and theoretical paradigms. The challenge is to reflect on them with a sceptical, uncertain and inquisitive stance, in order to open new possibilities with colleagues and generate a range of resources to apply to the situation they are seeking to help. Taking a community-oriented, psycho-social perspective enables staff to place a child and young person's behaviour in context, which can synthesise and evaluate all the potential explanations offered by other professionals.

Summary of key points

- As well as understanding why some children develop mental health problems, it is crucially important to learn more about those who in similar circumstances do not. Research is required to analyse the nature of these resilient children to understand whether coping strategies or skills can be transferred to others. Positive factors such as reduced social isolation, good schooling and supportive adults outside the family appear to help.

- Mental health problems can be distinguished by the term *disorder*, by the degree of seriousness and the length of time the condition lasts. The assumption is that most people will recognise these symptoms and understand they do not require specialist or intensive intervention.

- Research has revealed that GPs were only identifying 2 per cent of the 23 per cent of children attending surgeries who had some form of severe psychological or emotional problem (Freer, 2016). These findings are worrying because primary care is one of the most crucial gateways for troubled children and young people to gain access to appropriate services and resources and for signposting to accessible and acceptable support in this area.

- Understanding the key elements of human growth and development theoretical resources relevant to CAMHS is critical to social workers seeking to assess and intervene appropriately in the lives of troubled young people. Some social psychologists criticise the emphasis in child development theories on normative concepts and suggest enhancing the judging, measuring approach towards one that embodies context, culture and competencies.

✦ Linking child development with attachment theory can provide a sound theoretical knowledge base with which to assess a variety of situations you may encounter. An additional refinement would be to integrate systemic theory with attachment theory to enable a synthesis of the individual with the family context.

✦ Early childhood studies are beginning to challenge the orthodoxy in child development theories so that children are seen as accomplishing, living, competent persons rather than not yet quite fully formed people who are learning to become adults. The idea that the stages have to be accomplished sequentially ignores the different pace at which different children change according to external and other influences.

Further reading

Bryant-Waugh, R and Lask, B (2004) *Eating Disorders: A Parent's Guide*. London: Routledge.

Dendy, C (2006) *Teenagers with ADD and ADHD: A Guide for Parents and Professionals*. Bethesda, MD: Woodbine House.

Fonagy, P, Cottrell, D, Phillips, J, Bevington, D, Glaser, D and Allison, E (2016) *What Works for Whom? A Critical Review of Treatments for Children and Adolescents*. London: Guilford Press.

Prior, V and Glaser, D (2006) *Understanding Attachment and Attachment Disorders: Theory, Evidence, and Practice*. London: Jessica Kingsley.

Walker, S (2011) *The Social Worker's Guide to Child and Adolescent Mental Health*. London: Jessica Kingsley.

World Health Organization (2005) *Child and Adolescent Mental Health Policies and Plans*. Geneva: WHO.

✲ Internet resources

✲ NSPCC: **www.nspcc.org.uk**

✲ PAPYRUS – Prevention of Young Suicide: **www.papyrus-uk.org**

✲ Young People in Care: **www.becomecharity.org.uk**

Chapter 2: How to assess and understand young people

Introduction

Assessment is the starting point of any contact with troubled children and young people; therefore, it is a critical point in the journey of engaging with and helping them. Assessment has been defined as a tool to aid in the planning of future work and the beginning of helping the young person to identify areas for growth and change. Its purpose is the identification of needs – it is never an end in itself, although the process of assessment can of itself be therapeutic.

Assessment is the foundation on which to build a trusting relationship, which is the key to maximising the chance of a successful outcome. It can set the tone for further contact, it is your first opportunity to engage with a new or existing client, and it can be perceived by children and young people as a judgement on their character or behaviour. A good experience of assessment can make them feel positive about receiving help and their attitude to you and your agency. A bad experience of assessment can make matters worse, offend, and make problems harder to resolve in the long term. At worst it can be reduced to little more than a paper-chasing exercise, involving form-filling, an adherence to tick-box culture and participating in a process that restricts service eligibility. Or you can see it as an opportunity to engage with children and adolescents in a problem-solving partnership where both of you can learn more.

Principles underlying assessment

• **Critical thinking:** involves tapping into your natural curiosity; analysing underlying assumptions; considering multiple perspectives; reflecting; inquiring; and a certain amount of scepticism.

• **Knowledge:** a wide knowledge about the spectrum of problems that bring the public into contact with social services, eg in sexual abuse cases an understanding of child development, family systems, sex offenders, community resources, risk assessment, cultural dynamics and case management.

• **Principles of assessment:** recognise that using the principles of assessment alone may not provide assessment skills which are transferable to other settings and client groups.

• **Working in partnership:** crucial in working with troubled young people where social care, health and other professionals are mutually dependent on each other in the care assessment process.

The dimensions of a child's developmental needs

Health: growth, development, physical and mental well-being, genetic factors, disability, diet, exercise, immunisations, sex education, substance misuse.

Education: play and interaction, books, skills, interests, achievements, school, special educational needs.

Emotional and behavioural development: appropriateness of responses, expression of feelings, actions, attachments, temperament, adaptability, self-control, stress responses.

Identity: self-perception, abilities, self-image, self-esteem, individuality, race, religion, age, gender, sexuality, disability, sense of belonging, acceptance.

Family and social relationships: empathy, affectionate relationships, siblings, friendships.

Social presentation: appearance, behaviour, understanding of social self, dress, cleanliness, personal hygiene, use of advice.

Self-care skills: acquisition of competencies, independence, practical skills, confidence, problem-solving, vulnerabilities, impact of disability.

The dimensions of parenting capacity

Basic care: providing for physical needs, medical care, food, hygiene, warmth, shelter, clothing, hygiene.

Ensuring safety: protecting child from abuse, harm or danger, unsafe adults, self-harm, recognition of hazards.

Emotional warmth: meeting emotional needs, racial and cultural identity, valued, secure, stable and affectionate relationships, responsive to child's needs, praise, warm regard, encouragement and physical comfort.

Stimulation: cognitive stimulation, intellectual development, promoting social opportunities, interaction, communication, talking, encouraging questions, play, school attendance, enabling success.

Guidance and boundaries: help guide emotions and behaviour, demonstrating and modelling behaviour and interactions with others, setting boundaries, moral development, respect own values, anger management, consideration for others, discipline.

Stability: maintain secure attachments, consistent emotional warmth, predictable responses, maintain contact with other family members and significant others.

The dimensions of family and environmental factors

Family history and functioning: genetic and psycho-social factors, household composition, history of parent's own childhood, life events, family functioning, sibling relationships, parental strengths and difficulties, absent parents, separated parents' relationship.

Wider family: who does the child feel attached to? Related and non-related persons and wider family, role of relatives and friends, the importance of other people in family network.

Housing: amenities, accessibility, sanitation, cooking facilities, sleeping arrangements, hygiene, and safety.

Employment: who works, pattern of employment, meaning of work to the child, impact of work or absence of work on child.

Income: availability, sufficiency, welfare benefits, how resources are used, financial difficulties and the effect on the child.

Family's social integration: local neighbourhood, community, degree of integration or isolation, peer groups, friendships, social networks.

Community resources: local facilities and resources, health care, day care, schools, places of worship, transport, shops, leisure activities, standard of resources.

Appreciating strengths and difficulties

The complex interplay across all three domains should be carefully understood and analysed. The interactions between different factors within the domains are not straightforward. It is important then to gather and record information accurately and systematically. Information should be checked and discussed with parents and children. Differences in perceptions about the information and its relative significance should be recorded. It is important to assess and understand the strengths and difficulties within families and relate these to the vulnerabilities and protective factors in the child's world. The impact of what is happening on the child should be clearly identified.

A useful resource has been devised to incorporate a more positive view of assessment with children and adolescents. Staff can adapt this for use with parents to help empower them by understanding the detail of the problem and to focus on what needs to change. The Strengths and Difficulties Questionnaire addresses four areas of difficult behaviour: emotional symptoms, conduct problems, hyperactivity, and peer problems. It includes a prosocial behaviour (strengths) dimension to produce a numerical score with descriptions that are easy to recognise. One of its advantages is that professionals and parents/carers can use it to measure change in the child's behaviour before and after intervention. It therefore moves away from some of the more negative, deficit-oriented assessment instruments. Free copies of the questionnaire with background notes are available from www.youthinmind.com and further detailed information is available at www.sdqinfo.org. The Strengths and Difficulties Questionnaire (SDQ) is a brief behavioural screening questionnaire about 3 to 16 year olds. It exists in several versions to meet the needs of researchers, clinicians and educationalists. All versions of the SDQ ask about 25 attributes, some positive and others negative. These 25 items are divided between five scales:

- emotional symptoms (five items);

- conduct problems (five items);

- hyperactivity/inattention (five items);

- peer relationship problems (five items);

- prosocial behaviour (five items).

The same 25 items are included in questionnaires for completion by the parents or teachers of 4 to 16 year olds. There is a slightly modified informant-rated version for the parents or nursery teachers of 3 and 4 year olds: 22 items are identical, the item on reflectiveness is softened, and two items on anti-social behaviour are replaced by items on oppositionality. Questionnaires for self-completion by adolescents ask about the same 25 traits, though the wording is slightly different. This self-report version is suitable for young people aged around 11 to 16, depending on their level of understanding and literacy.

✎ Activity 2.1

🔦 Review the above information and consider what makes sense to you or confirms ideas you already hold.

🔦 Consider adapting these ideas into your own practice, and perhaps adding some that are new to you.

💬 Commentary

These models are not mutually exclusive; rather, they can work together or in sequence depending on the age and stage of the child's development. A health visitor, youth worker, community police officer, school nurse or CAMHS worker may identify other risk factors in the community, or if similar, they might rank them in a different order of priority concern. While there are a number of specific protective factors, these may vary over time depending on the child's age and resources available.

What are the early warning signs of mental health problems?

The charity Action for Children have come up with a checklist – aided by a useful mnemonic MASK – to help spot early signs that may be leading to a young person developing mental health problems (Action for Children, 2019). Young people will naturally go through huge emotional changes and mood swings during puberty and adolescence. For some individuals these may be prolonged and low intensity and for others they may be short-lived and high intensity. But if the following are happening at the same time then an assessment is indicated:

M – MOOD

They get irritable, argumentative or aggressive towards you. They may blame you if things go wrong. They can also become withdrawn.

A – ACTIONS

They may experience changes in eating and sleeping patterns. Look out for any signs of bullying, alcohol, drugs or self-harm.

S – SOCIAL

They suddenly appear especially bored, lonely or withdrawn or they start to get into trouble. Losing interest in friends and other things they liked to do or missing school are common warning signs.

K – KEEP TALKING

Refusing or being reluctant to talk about how they're feeling is common. But keep listening and ask how they are feeling. When they do open up, make sure they know there's someone there who really cares.

What is the role of stress and threat and the propensity to develop mental health problems?

Many researchers (including Rodway et al, 2016) highlight the impact of severe and prolonged stress and difficulty on young people's psycho-social and psychological development across a wide range of functions. Children can feel threatened in different ways: events may threaten their sense of who they are (identity and status), of what they can do (self-efficacy, self-esteem) and their physical or emotional security (when events or people are unpredictable and their behaviour is intimidating or threatening). Young children will feel these uncertainties more intensely, partly because they are more dependent and need to rely on patterns, routines and parents to help them feel safe and cared for.

It is also partly because their sense of self is emergent, and therefore not robust, and partly because they cannot easily anticipate change, imagine how they will cope or know from experience how things can improve over time. Children find many ingenious ways to neutralise their fears and protect their self-respect (such as lying and cheating, being disruptive and not listening). Some of these responses can be seen as 'difficult' or not in their longer-term interest and can start a pattern of behaviour that becomes increasingly dysfunctional, off-putting and abnormal.

How much does food and diet affect behaviour and emotional well-being?

There is considerable public and professional interest in what role food has in mitigating mental health problems or in exacerbating a latent predisposition. But focusing exclusively on food and diet is inadequate in pursuing solutions to multiple and complex emotional and mental health problems in young people. There is growing interest in the effect of diet on behaviour in the national debate on school dinners, but nutritional improvements in one meal a day only during term time will not be a panacea for dealing with classroom disruption. Naturally, hungry children will concentrate less well, as will those fired up on sugar.

Those not receiving essential nutrients may be more impulsive or think more slowly, and mood, application and thinking processes may improve when recommended proportions of fatty acids are present in the diet. Dietary improvements could have an exponential effect on learning, given that much learning is incremental, and could help children to 'catch up' optimally on some aspects of development during periods of neural plasticity, when the brain is programmed to be receptive to stimuli and restructure.

In addition, if the debate also encourages families to cook more fresh food and eat together more frequently, this could help children to feel more cared for, and so raise their confidence and competence further. Nevertheless, it is hard to see how diet might offset totally the effects of early and prolonged harsh discipline, serial family disruption, trauma or neglect. Disruptive behaviour has many different causes because young children have few ways to express complex feelings such as frustration, boredom, anger, fear, dejection, jealousy and a need for attention. Some equally troubled children become excessively quiet and diligent, and these should not be ignored. Multiple causes demand multiple interventions.

What are the general risk factors for developing mental health problems?

Over recent decades, professionals have become increasingly aware of and concerned about the physical and psychological effect of abuse on children, especially sexual abuse, more latterly physical abuse and, to a lesser extent, emotional abuse (as a consequence of neglect). Largely because prolonged and serious neglect is now rare, tends to occur behind closed doors and any damage may not show immediately, it has not been easy to conduct research. But if neglect at home persists, even if it is less severe, the cumulative damage may become significant. The term *mentalisation* has been used to describe the capacity to interpret the behaviour of others (and oneself) in terms of mental states (beliefs, wishes, feelings, desires) – in short, the ability to recognise that other people have minds. The experience of both trauma and neglect inhibit the natural development of this capacity because the individual reverts to a more infantile state of mental functioning.

Neglect is different from trauma in that trauma relates to an event while emotional neglect characterises the relationship and tends to be ongoing. During early brain development, there are sensitive periods during which particular experiences dovetail with pre-programmed stages of brain maturation. The complex interconnections between different areas of the brain, each with its own timetable for critical periods of maturation, contribute to the varied outcomes and developmental complications of early detrimental experiences. For infants, some developments require particular environmental influences, such as safe handling, responsive gaze and intimate talking.

From the available research, the conclusion is that neglect and failure of environmental stimulation during critical periods of brain development may lead to permanent deficits in cognitive abilities (Walker, 2011a). The infant brain is programmed to expect stimuli to be presented in a 'safe, nurturing, predictable, repetitive, gradual' way, attuned to the developmental stage (Walker, 2011a, p 260). The right kind of sensitive attention also helps the caregiver to regulate the infant's arousal and impulses, to help cope with, often intense, frustration. The next activity will prompt you to understand that external factors are as important as internal factors in assessing children and young people who may be or are at risk of becoming mentally ill.

✎ Activity 2.2

🖊 Spend time reflecting on the community and families you work with; highlight both the general and the environmentally specific factors which may lead to children and young people being at risk.

🖊 Would this list contain different risk factors if a colleague from a different agency or organisation undertook this activity?

💬 Commentary

When exploring the record you have compiled, it is worth remembering that this is a potential list. Some children and families may live through and survive emotional, physical or financial trauma with their family life intact, while other families may not be able to endure relatively minor changes in family circumstances. This can be due to a number of resilience factors an individual or family may have. Studies which have investigated the concept define resilience 'as an end product or buffering process that does not eliminate risks and stress but that allows the individual to deal with them effectively'. There are three main mechanisms which enable these protective factors to occur.

• **Compensation:** offers a framework where stress and protective factors counterbalance each other and personal qualities and support can outweigh the stress.

• **Challenge as a protective mechanism:** highlights the strength that a moderate amount of stress can add to levels of competence.

• **Immunity:** the protective factors within the child or their environment moderate the impact of the stress on the child, and the child adapts to the changing environment with less trauma.

What are the concerns of young people?

Researchers have interviewed young people (Children's Commissioner, 2018) and discovered children and young people wished to:

- be fit and well;

- feel protected and secure;

- enjoy pleasurable experiences;

- reach their potential ability;

- give something back to society;

- not be poor.

One of the enduring problems for staff is encountering children and young people who from many experiences feel they will not be believed or that it is wrong to disclose abuse happening to them. Thus they will not open up until and unless the right conditions are created to enable them to share distressing information or details. The latest government school exclusion figures show that there were about 1,000 more permanent exclusions in the year 2015–16 (6,685 exclusions in all) than there were the year before (The Guardian, 2017b). That's out of a total of the roughly 8 million children attending state schools in England. It works out as eight in every 10,000 primary and secondary school pupils, up from seven in every 10,000 the previous year. Until recently, overall exclusion numbers had continued to fall. This could be interpreted as a measure of success in keeping children in school, indicating improved behaviour and potentially fewer mental health issues. On the other hand, evidence suggests that league table sensitivity, Ofsted reports and other indicators demonstrate a less clear picture. Schools can juggle the concept of exclusion to influence the numbers permanently excluded, temporarily or even internally excluded from lessons.

This is why certain pupils, such as those from Irish Traveller or black Caribbean communities or with special educational needs, remain over-represented in school exclusions. The consequences of being permanently excluded from school matter enormously for any child. For example, 40 per cent of 16 to 18 year olds not in education, employment or training (NEETS) have been permanently excluded (The Guardian, 2017b). According to Her Majesty's Inspectorate of Prisons (2017), nine out of ten incarcerated young people who had offended were excluded from school before the age of 14 and never re-engaged. This emphasises again the need for a systemic, sustainable approach to be applied across and within agencies who have been corralled into their own separate, isolated system by structural and financial constraints preventing inter-agency communication.

How can risk factors for abuse and individual circumstances of the young person be considered?

While physical, emotional or sexual abuse is a concern for every child and young person with regard to their individual experiences, it is more complex as the effects of abuse are influenced by other factors. The type of association between the child and the abuser will have an impact. Most abuse is perpetrated by someone known to the young person such as a family member, relative or friend. For example, if the child sees the person every day and consequently develops a constant fear of abuse, this may be more harmful than a child who sees their abuser infrequently. When the abuse is brutal, it could be more damaging than if the abuse is perceived as more restrained.

The child's age and developmental stage have to also be taken into consideration. It may be that a young person who already has a clear picture of who they are may be less affected by abuse, no matter how severe, compared to a young child who is still discovering their own self-worth and value. Finally, it could be that the duration of the abuse and how often the abuse occurs may also have a bearing on the long-term outcome for the child or young person. However, each child and young person is unique and their level of resilience to the effects of abuse will also be individual to them. This is an area of great uncertainty calling for a capacity in the worker to 'hold' this uncertainty and the anxiety that accompanies it. This can only be done through constant reflective practice and sophisticated supervision skills.

A young person who is sexually abused will require considerable support and care if they ever summon the courage to disclose what has happened to them. Teachers are often the person chosen by the young person, probably because they are a constant figure, trusted and not part of their family. In the course of supporting such a young person displaying signs of mental health problems, a counsellor might also be told the truth about what happened as a precursor to the start of the mental health problems. Professionals working in this highly sensitive area know that the child protection and safeguarding procedures can often adversely impact therapeutic work. From experience, they also know that legal proceedings against a perpetrator can fail to proceed based on the age of the young person, their perceived competence to give evidence in court and the reduced likelihood of securing a conviction without forensic or corroborative evidence.

Risk assessment and risk management strategies

The evidence suggests that interplay between characteristics in the child and their environment increases the risks of developing mental health problems. Workers ought to find this paradigm fits with a holistic psycho-social framework for assessment and intervention. The rise in drug and substance abuse, alcohol consumption and the widening gap between rich and poor all contribute to a fertile environment for risk factors to escalate. The risks to children from parents with mental health problems are well understood, yet there is still evidence of a lack of liaison between adult and child and adolescent mental health services, which would better serve all the family members.

Genetic versus environmental mediation studies show that both parental education and parental depression influence the likelihood of mental health outcomes for children, and in both, the genetic effect will be mediated by the environment. Preventive and predictive risk assessment aims to target support services early enough to reach those most in need. However, this process can be discriminatory, inaccurate and statistically unreliable. Poor families and socially excluded people can feel persecuted. Checklists of predictive factors have led to the construction of characteristics of parents more likely to harm their children. They imply that it is only in socially disadvantaged families where abuse is more likely to take place, or that single parents, those abused in childhood, or fostered and adopted children are likely to abuse their own children. This is inaccurate, unhelpful and potentially dangerous.

✎ Activity 2.3

🔍 Obtain a copy of your agency guidelines on risk assessment in relation to children's mental health.

🔍 After consulting it, reflect with a colleague on its strengths and weaknesses.

💬 Commentary

The evidence for the effectiveness of risk assessments is not reassuring. A study of risk assessment models in the United States which mirror principles enshrined in UK guidance found that there was too high a rate of error in them, and that staff tended to standardise practice at the expense of employing wider risk assessment methods. The current norms of risk assessment are still based on a white, middle-class, gendered ideology. The tools of risk assessment tend not to take account of cultural factors in their construction or interpretation. There is considerable pressure on staff and their managers to make safe decisions, which can be judged as such before and after the event. Such an impossible task leads to defensive practice and the neglect of child mental health problems, which are difficult to quantify.

Resilience factors to mitigate mental health problems

Children with several identified risk factors demonstrate resilience and do not develop mental health problems. As well as understanding why some children develop mental health problems, it is crucially important to learn more about those who in similar circumstances do not. Research is required to analyse the nature of these resilient children to understand whether coping strategies or skills can be transferred to other children. Positive factors such as reduced social isolation, good schooling and supportive adults outside the family appear to help. These are the very factors missing in asylum seekers, refugees and other ethnic minority families who live in deprived conditions and suffer more socio-economic disadvantages than other children.

Resilience is an important theoretical concept as it encompasses the complexity of causal factors. It acknowledges, for example, the influence of both social and environmental factors and individual differences, and identifies what helps individuals to cope and what increases the risk that they will not. It also accepts that a particular, perhaps unexpected, event, when added to other earlier or concurrent difficulties apparently coped with, can trigger a behavioural or emotional crisis, while as an isolated event it may not have done so. Resilience arises out of a belief in one's own sense of agency, the ability to deal with change and a repertoire of social and problem-solving skills.

Having a sense of agency and a coherent narrative of personal history that makes sense of the world are both necessary for the formation of a sound identity. The resilience framework does not, however, address causation in depth. This raises a danger that the associated protective and risk factors are given undue prominence in policy, with the more telling underlying causal factors or relationships, contextual influences and implications insufficiently appreciated. Personal characteristics that protect individuals (secure attachment, average to high intelligence, good communication, planning and problem-solving skills, humour, reflective capacity, religious faith and easy temperament) are largely interrelated.

A secure attachment will encourage easy communication, reflection and, because the future (based on past experience) feels safe, the inclination to think ahead, sequence actions, plan and develop a 'can-do' approach to anticipated problems. If a child is not securely attached, they are more likely to feel that their very sense of self is under threat. Living in and for the moment, they will have little room for reflection, and consequently less space to feel concern for others (which is crucially important for the development of a rounded and whole personality).

🖉 Activity 2.4

🢔 What are the key factors that promote resilience in young people to mental health problems and disorders?

🗩 Commentary

Factors within the young person include:

• the child's response to stress being determined by the capacity to appraise and attach meaning to their situation;

• age-related susceptibilities which permit older children to use their greater understanding compared to younger children;

• how a child deals with adversity either actively or reactively; the ability to act positively is a function of self-esteem and feelings of self-efficacy rather than of any inherent problem-solving skills;

• the quality of a child's resilience to developing mental health problems or emotional and behavioural difficulties is influenced by early life experiences but is not determinative of later outcomes.

Mental health problems frequently present in children and young people who are causing concern to staff working in education, social services or in youth justice contexts. The capability of teachers, social workers and probation officers, and the capacity of the services within which they work to identify these mental health problems, are crucial. Key factors promoting resilience are: self-esteem, sociability and autonomy; family compassion, warmth, an absence of parental discord; and social support systems that encourage personal effort and coping. Being able to respond in a timely and appropriate manner to the early signs of mental health problems may make all the difference to the chance of effective intervention for the young person. There remain, however, barriers to the development of wider and better understanding of mental health difficulties among and between professionals in all agencies coming into contact with troubled children. These include:

- a widespread reluctance to 'label' a child or young person as mentally ill;

- a poor appreciation of what specialist child psychology and psychiatry services can do;

- the ways in which priorities are set within the statutory framework of the Mental Health Act 1983, Children Act 1989 and the Education Act 1993;

- lack of knowledge and close working between agencies.

What is holistic assessment?

Assessment methodology in specialist child and adolescent mental health services tends to remain rooted in psychiatric diagnostic models with psycho-social factors included as risk factors reflecting negative, deficit indicators. Workers need to embrace a more holistic approach seeking to identify and amplify strengths, coping strategies, alternative community resources and user perceptions. It has been established that a confluence of several risk factors in childhood can create the conditions for later psycho-social difficulty, including socio-economic disadvantage, child abuse and parental mental illness. However, there are protective mechanisms that can mitigate the chance of some children going on to develop anti-social behaviour or serious mental health problems.

A thorough assessment of risk *and* resilience factors is advocated. These include the child's response to stress being determined by the capacity to appraise and attach meaning to their situation. Age-related susceptibilities that permit older children to use their greater understanding compared to younger children need to be understood. How a child deals with adversity either actively or reactively, and the ability to act positively, is a function of self-esteem and feelings of self-efficacy rather than indicating any inherent problem-solving skills. Features as varied as secure, stable and affectionate relationships, success, achievement and temperamental attributes can foster such cognitive capacity.

These personal qualities seem to be operative as much in their effects on interactions with and responses from other people, as in their role in regulating individual responses to life events. Coping successfully with stressful situations can be a strengthening experience and promotes resilience, which can allow self-confidence to increase. Protection does not necessarily lie in the buffering effects of some supportive factor. Rather, all the evidence points towards the importance of developmental links. The quality of a child's resilience to developing mental health problems or emotional and behavioural difficulties is influenced by early life experiences but is not determinative of later outcomes.

This highlights the importance of assessment methods that take account of not just individual characteristics within the child but equally within the family and broader environment. In combination, these protective factors may create a chain of indirect links that foster escape from adversity. Organising services across the spectrum of multi-agency provision in partnership between social work professionals and parents offers the opportunity to bring out dormant protective factors to interrupt the causal chain of negative events. A progressive, preventive environment that promotes children's emotional well-being is preferable to reacting to the consequences of neglect or abuse.

Individual factors regarded as promoting resilience include:

- an even and adaptable temperament;

- a capacity for problem-solving;

- physical attractiveness;

- a sense of humour;

- good social skills and supportive peers;

- a sense of autonomy and purpose;

- secure attachment to at least one parent;

- links with the wider community.

✎ Activity 2.5 Case illustration

Freddy is 14 years old with mild learning disabilities and has been diagnosed with autism. He lives with his father and younger brother, who is 12 years old. Freddy's father has declined an offer of respite care to give him a break from the stress of caring for the family. A friend helps out sometimes by taking Freddy and his brother to the local gym, but Freddy is becoming more and more withdrawn, particularly since his mother left the family home. He was assessed for a place at a special school for children with autism but his parents could not agree on the matter and he is now in a local school where they try hard to include Freddy but are finding him a handful. He has extra support in class and his teacher has received advice from educational psychologists and the National Autistic Society. Freddy finds it difficult to cope, however. He has been involved in fights with other boys and when he is not allowed to continue with his favourite activity of painting he has become aggressive towards teaching staff. He has no friends at school and his reading and writing are five years behind his peers. Freddy has been referred to your social work team. Your task is to assess the situation and come up with a plan of action.

💬 Commentary

Assessment

Freddy needs to be understood in the context of his family and social environment. His behaviour needs to be seen as a means of communicating his distress, which he cannot express in other ways. You need to be aware that his reported behaviours can be due to emotional problems rather than assume they are an integral feature of autism. Remember that Freddy is at a developmental transition into adolescence and his behaviours may be associated with this life stage, similar to his peers. However, Freddy will be aware that his peers have abilities he does not. The school environment may not be fully understanding or supportive of his needs. At home, his father could be finding Freddy difficult to cope with now he is physically larger and stronger, but his pride causes him to resist offers of help. He is unsure about how to advise Freddy about his sexuality and curiosity about intimate relationships.

Intervention

Close observation of Freddy in school and at home together with other professional assessments will provide rich information for you to evaluate. The core aim of your intervention is to facilitate his communication and help improve the physical environments in order to provide Freddy with a degree of predictability. It is important that he can exit situations where he is over-stimulated and can retire to a safe, calm space to unwind. Individual behavioural interventions can be helpful for use in the school or home setting so that he can gain positive feedback when keeping on task. Freddy might also require counselling/therapeutic input to address anxiety problems underlying some of his troubling behaviours.

Overall educational provision may need to be reviewed to assess whether existing plans require updating or changing to reflect his emerging needs. His father will probably benefit from some individual support from you to discuss his feelings about Freddy and the break-up of the marriage. Provision of good quality information about autism could help his father gain further insight and empathy with Freddy's behaviour and future care needs. You could assume the role of keyworker in co-ordinating planning and arranging multi-agency meetings with the family to foster collaborative and empowering relationships.

⚒ Summary of key points

✦ Children vary in their vulnerability to psycho-social stress and adversity as a result of both genetic and environmental influences. Family-wide experiences tend to impinge on individual children in quite different ways. The reduction of negative chain reactions and increase of positive chain reactions influence the extent to which the effects of adversity persist over time.

✦ New experiences that open up opportunities can provide beneficial turning-point effects. Although positive experiences in themselves do not exert much of a protective effect, they can be helpful if they serve to neutralise some risk factors, and the cognitive and affective processing of experiences is likely to be a positive influence whether or not resilience develops.

✦ Evidence-based practice requires the gathering, testing, recording and weighing of evidence on which to base decisions and the careful use of knowledge gained during culturally competent assessment work with a child and family.

✦ The critical task is determining what is most relevant in a family's situation, what is most significant for the child, the impact intervention is having, and the judgement about when more or less action is required in the child's best interests. It is important to pay equal attention to all three domains and not be deflected by a child's emotional or behavioural symptoms to the extent that parental capacity and environmental factors are neglected.

✦ Assessments can become dominated by the agenda of particular agencies when issues of protection or neglect are at stake, thereby undermining the concept of inter-agency co-operation. Another factor is the drive to complete recording forms within specified timescales, culturally competent practice is given a lack of attention, while the pace of the assessment is inconsistent with the capacity of the family to cope.

✦ All staff working with troubled young people have a crucial role to play in engaging with other agencies where anxieties can tumble out of control in the climate of stress, blame and persecution surrounding their practice. A thoughtful, reflective intervention in the context of case conferences or agency meetings combined with insights developed in culturally competent work can go a long way to mitigate or contain potentially destructive processes.

Further reading

Carr-Gregg, N and Shale, E (2003) *Adolescence: A Guide for Parents*. London: Random House.

Fitzpatrick, C and Sharry, J (2004) *Coping with Depression in Young People: A Guide for Parents*. London: Wiley.

Goodman, A and Goodman, R (2012) Strengths and Difficulties Questionnaire Scores and Mental Health in Looked After Children. *The British Journal of Psychiatry*, 200: 426–7.

Parkin, A, Warner-Gale, F, Frake, G and Dogra, N (2017) *A Multidisciplinary Handbook of Child and Adolescent Mental Health for Front-line Professionals* (3rd ed). London: Jessica Kingsley.

Pike, R (2017) *Autism: Talking about a Diagnosis*. London: National Autistic Society.

Thapar, A, Pine, D S, Leckman, J F, Scott, S, Snowling, M J and Taylor, E A (2015) *Rutter's Child and Adolescent Psychiatry* (6th ed). London: Wiley Blackwell.

Internet resources

Assessment: **www.rcpsych.ac.uk**

National Centre for Eating Disorders: **www.eating-disorders.org.uk**

National Children's Bureau: **www.ncb.org.uk**

Chapter 3: Why are diversity, cultural awareness and social inclusion important?

Introduction

There is now an established body of research demonstrating that Black, Asian and minority ethnic communities have higher diagnosed rates of mental health problems than the general population (Bhui and McKenzie, 2008). Disproportionate numbers of young black men are being labelled as mentally ill and subjected to restrictive or medication-based treatment. There is a pressing need to include the experience of service users and carers from black and ethnic minority communities to ensure help is appropriate and acceptable. In addition to the needs of black and ethnic minority children and young people being neglected, these findings also represent the institutionalisation of fear of 'the Other'.

The idea of 'otherness' is central to analyses of how majority and minority identities are constructed. This is because the representation of different groups within any given society is controlled by groups that have greater political power. In order to understand the notion of 'the Other', it is important to first seek to put a critical eye on the ways in which social identities are constructed. Rather than talking about the individual characteristics or personalities of different individuals, it is more useful to consider young people as having social identities. Social identities reflect the way in which individuals and groups internalise established social categories within their societies, such as their cultural (or ethnic) identities, gender identities, class identities and sexual identities. These social categories shape our ideas about who we think we are, how we want to be seen by others, and the groups to which we belong.

Understanding Black, Asian and minority ethnic families

In seeking to understand more, you need to be able to review the social context of mental health, cultural variations in emotional expression, and the wider effects of racism in producing higher levels of stress and disadvantage among black and ethnic minority children and young people. This is additionally compounded by practices in psychiatric services that are perceived to be institutionally racist and insensitive to individual needs. The development of psychiatry and theories of human growth and development constructed in the eighteenth and nineteenth centuries were based on white ethnocentric beliefs and assumptions about normality. The Western model of illness regards the mind as distinct from the body and defines mental illness or mental health according to negative, deficit characteristics. In non-Western cultures such as Chinese, Indian and African cultures, mental health is often perceived as a harmonious balance between a person's internal and external influences. Thus a person is intrinsically linked to their environment and vice versa.

The Western model of assessment of mental illness tends to ignore the religious or spiritual aspects of the culture in which it is based. However, Eastern, African and Native American cultures tend to integrate them. Spirituality and religion as topics in general do not feature often in the clinical literature, yet they can be critical components of a young person's well-being, offering a source of strength and hope in trying circumstances. Clients for whom family and faith backgrounds are inseparable may need encouragement to feel comfortable in multi-faith settings. You need to address this dimension as part of the constellation of factors affecting black children and young people, bearing in mind the positive and sometimes negative impact spiritual or religious beliefs might have on their mental health. It is also important to recognise that children do not have one essential identity, but switch identities in different situations and, subject to a diversity of cultural influences, can produce new identities.

This is the case with black and Asian children and young people influenced by the cultural norms of their white peers, while feeling pressured to maintain religious or cultural practices from elders. Employing anti-racist and anti-discriminatory principles may simplistically try to reinforce apparent cultural norms which are not applicable, or explain disturbed behaviour in terms of cultural features which are irrelevant or miss emerging mental health problems. A children's rights model of practice offers staff the resources to maintain anti-racist principles working with established black communities as well as insights into the inner world of refugee and asylum-seeking children and adolescents traumatised by war, ethnic persecution and profound losses.

Perceptions of child and adolescent problems

Practitioners seeking to assess, plan and intervene effectively with children and adolescents from diverse cultures have to carefully consider the various ways potential mental health problems are thought about, understood and communicated in every family, in every culture. In particular, the following points should be kept in mind.

• Children do not have one essential identity, but switch identities in different situations and, subject to a diversity of cultural influences, can produce new identities.

• Practitioners employing anti-racist and anti-discriminatory principles may simplistically try to reinforce apparent cultural norms that are not applicable, or explain disturbed behaviour in terms of cultural features which are irrelevant.

- Understanding the culture within the culture – in other words, finding out what are the individual and family norms, preferences, styles, habits and patterns of relationships that make that family what it is in the particular context of psychological problems.

For example, there is an assumption that Asian families are close-knit with extended family relationships often living together in multi-generational households. This is a stereotype and while it may apply to a lot of Asian families the danger is in applying the stereotype unthinkingly instead of using it to test a hypothesis about the particular family being helped. In many circumstances, taking into account the concept of extended family relationships in close proximity can aid assessment of emerging mental health problems in an Asian child or young person. But assuming this is *always* a sign of family strength and harmonious supportive relationships is risking missing obscure, destructive dynamics that may be contributing to the child's mental health problems. These factors are beginning to emerge as some Asian youth struggle to balance loyalty to their history and culture with the different values and pressures in their modern, Western environment.

A failure to recognise and acknowledge significant mental health problems could be just as damaging to the young person and others involved with them, as could seeking to explain their behaviour with a definitive psychiatric diagnosis. For some young people it could be a relief to have an explanation for feelings and behaviour that they find hard to make sense of, whereas for others it could exacerbate feelings of blame, guilt and self-loathing. The enduring social stigma of mental health problems in addition to racist experiences provides an overall context for these feelings to be repressed, displaced or acted out.

Very little of the research on the mental health consequences of black and other ethnic minority children witnessing domestic violence has examined the impact that race and racism might have on these children. It has been suggested that the societal context of racism provides these children with a sense of refuge inside their own home. However, when violence occurs inside their home as well, this can have profound effects on the child's sense of security and vulnerability, triggering acute anxiety-related symptoms. For these children there is no hiding place. Some of the negative impacts on black children are likely to be exacerbated by additional threats of abduction abroad, and/or by being asked inappropriately to act as interpreters or translators in situations where their protection is at stake.

✎ Activity 3.1

Consider in what ways Black, Asian and ethnic minority young people are excluded and their cultures negated by the majority dominant ideas.

💬 Commentary

In a postcolonial world, the rights and expectations of Indigenous people to reparation and how they are perceived are important issues in the context of achieving culturally competent practice. The disparities between developed and developing economies under the influence of globalisation are becoming more pronounced, incorporating new forms of cultural domination. The concept of cultural and social injustice can be illustrated thus:

> **Cultural domination:** some young people are excluded because they are subjected to ways of interpreting or communicating which originate from a culture which is not their own, and which may be alien or hostile to them.

> **Non-recognition:** some young people are excluded because they are effectively rendered invisible by the dominant cultural practices.

> **Cultural disrespect:** some young people are excluded because they are routinely devalued by the stereotyping of public representations or everyday interactions within the dominant cultural context.

What is the impact of racism on young people's mental health?

The impact of institutional and personal racism is difficult to measure or assess accurately because of its cumulative nature; however, it can result in a decreased sense of optimism, displaced anger and a retreat into individualism for survival of the spirit. Constant victimisation and exploitation result in rage and conflicts between self-realisation and the restrictions imposed by membership of a minority group. The sense of limited control over external social realities and subsequent feelings of helplessness and powerlessness lead to depression. Black and other ethnic minority young women face a double disadvantage in a racist and patriarchal society where they attract the projected hate of those white women and black men who are subordinated to white men.

In the context of holistic planning, it is important to understand how public perceptions of mental health problems are organised in a multi-cultural society. In addition, the ethnicity and gender of the client and clinician are critical variables influencing diagnosis. High frequencies of psychosis and low frequencies of depression are diagnosed in black populations combined with stereotyped perceptions that ethnic minority children and young people have less insight than their white counterparts.

How can help for black young people be made more accessible?

The characteristics of a service for black children and adolescents with mental health problems which aspires to better accessibility can be described as consisting of three elements:

Consultation with individual black families and their communities is required to ensure service provision meets their needs and to identify gaps in services. A pro-active community-oriented practice offers a practical and effective way of achieving this.

Information needs to be provided about rights and responsibilities in the context of childcare and mental health legislation. Jargon-free material should be accessible in different formats and languages about child and adolescent mental health needs.

Competence – staff competence in child and adolescent mental health is not enough if this is not matched with demonstrable knowledge and skills required to practise in an ethnically diverse society.

How important is religion and spirituality?

An increasingly diverse, multicultural and ethnically rich society is enabling a wider understanding of the cultural characteristics of modern Britain. For young people's mental health these are important factors to consider. Four core qualities of spiritual experience have been identified in young people: awareness, mystery, value, and meaningfulness/insight. They are often assumed to be consistent with positive life-affirming experiences. However, children who experience wonder, awe and mystery can quickly become distressed and fearful – even terrified – if a secure and stable main carer is not available to contain those negative feelings.

Many religions contain concepts of hell and punishment which could trigger profound feelings of despair that are experienced as completely overwhelming both physically and psychologically. Research with young people has revealed that while many don't have an active religious belief system, most have a sense of spirituality (Walker, 2010). When this is explored it means that they have a sense of something intangible beyond themselves, which causes feelings of awe and wonder. Popular scientific TV programmes and documentaries which explore concepts of time, the creation of life and how big the universe is can seem hard to fathom but also instil a feeling of amazement and overwhelming emotions.

Discussing these ideas with young people can offer the opportunity to place themselves in a much wider context than everyday worries or particular stressful situations. A sense of wonder can help encourage deep attention, positive feelings, changes in behaviour, and combined with curiosity can help a troubled young person feel good and connect to phenomena beyond themselves. We live in an age of distraction, hyper-communication, individualisation and 24-hour information as well as a coarsening of personal debate and public discourse. Young people are at the centre of this vortex and all the evidence is that it is harming them mentally.

Sin is defined variously in many religions and for a child or young person comes with the sense of failing to be satisfactory – for example from early toileting experiences through to exam performance or adolescent sexuality. The sense of sin and failure is quickly transformed into guilt and shame, resulting in feelings of depression, distress and despair unless there is some balancing influence. Children and young people without this balancing experience and with deficits in their environment and personal temperament are likely to develop mental health problems at the time or later on in life. It is easy for children to feel that they are failing or cannot fit easily into the world. This is the opposite of spiritual experiences of value, insight and relatedness. A persistent sense of sinfulness or failure prevents the development of healthy relationships.

Therapy and cultural belief

Some young people may believe that their problem(s) are the result of divine intervention – a punishment for a sin or misdemeanour of some kind. Among some cultures there is a potent belief system that spirits can possess people and make them unwell or be invoked to help them with a problem. In the case of a child or young person who is causing concern among teachers, social workers or health professionals, there may be a simple diagnosis or assessment of the cause of the problem but this may not fit with the family's beliefs about the cause. However, belief also relates to religion and spirituality. If the therapist is unable or unwilling to explore this aspect of belief then they may be missing a vital component of the individual or family's overall belief system about how the world works and how problems arise, and more importantly what is likely to be effective treatment.

In order to respond to this context, workers seeking to harness positive aspects of religion and spirituality in their work, a theory of multicultural therapy has been advanced that offers a multidimensional paradigm to guide intervention with these key elements.

- Both worker and young person identities are formed and embedded in multiple levels of life experiences and contexts; therefore, support should take greater account of the child or young person's experience in relation to their context.

- The cultural identity development of the worker and young person, and the wider power differentials associated with this, play an important role in the helping relationship.

- Multicultural counselling and therapy effectiveness is enhanced when the worker uses flexible methods and defines goals consistent with the life experiences and cultural values of the young person.

✏ Activity 3.2

✎ Discuss with a colleague or friend what are the advantages of multicultural counselling and therapy.
✎ Consider ways in which your support and the service you work in could improve in this area.

💬 Commentary

Multicultural counselling and therapy helps the child or young person develop a greater awareness about themselves in relation to their different contexts. This results in support that is contextual in orientation and able to respectfully draw on traditional methods of healing with a spiritual or religious dimension from many cultures. It is perhaps a paradox that the decline of organised religion in white Western societies, combined with the consequences of previous imperialist expansion throughout the world, has produced a growing culturally diverse population among whom are large numbers of devout religious communities with highly developed spiritual belief systems that organise social behaviour.

While pundits, politicians and policy makers observe increases in anti-social behaviour among disaffected and disadvantaged young white people and blame the absence of religious values and thus moral standards, they are at the same time witnessing a growth in ethnic minority religious and spiritual affiliation resulting in social, psychological and educational attainment. Culturally competent practice aspires to understand and support both groups of children and young people to help them make sense of their beliefs or lack of them in terms of vulnerability or resistance to psychological problems.

Children and young people with learning disabilities

Children and adolescents with learning disabilities are over six times more likely to have a diagnosable psychiatric disorder than their peers who do not have learning disabilities. Around half of those young people had received no help from specialist CAMHS teams. Recent research from Emerson and Hatton (2007) shows that 39 per cent of 5 to 15 year-old British children with learning disabilities had a diagnosable mental health problem (compared to 8 per cent among children who did not have learning disabilities). It has been found that they are more likely to:

• be boys, have poor general health and fewer friends;

• have been exposed to a greater variety of adverse life events (eg abuse, serious accidents, bereavement, domestic violence);

• be brought up by a single parent (nearly always a single mother);

• live in poverty and a poorly functioning family;

• have a mother who is in poorer health and has mental health needs;

• live in a family with lower educational attainment and higher rates of unemployment.

What are the implications?

Considerable social disadvantage is faced by children with learning disabilities and their families. All of the above have also been identified as risk factors for mental health problems among children and adolescents generally. What this means is that we would expect children with learning disabilities to have more mental health problems, not as an inevitable consequence of their learning disabilities, but simply because of their increased chances of being exposed to poverty, social exclusion and more challenging family environments.

Children and young people with a learning disability are currently supposed to receive mental health services in a variety of settings, including not only traditional CAMHS but also community paediatric services, child development centres, specialist learning disability (LD) services and special needs educational services. The co-ordination of care between these services is variable nationally. Only 49 per cent of CAMHS services were recently reported as being accessible to children and young people with learning disabilities (Emerson and Hatton, 2007). Improving access to CAMHS for children with learning disabilities has been a key national target in recent years and yet again appeared in the latest CAMHS review as a major limitation in current service provision (Walker, 2016).

This reflects a long history of neglect of these vulnerable socially excluded young people. Until very recently, service provision consisted of a policy of normalisation based on individualised care, behaviour modification strategies and an overall medicalised view of their needs. Any psychological or therapeutic needs were largely denied. Statutory and voluntary services have developed unhelpful dichotomies between learning disability and mental health services. This results in children and young people with mental health problems and learning disabilities falling between the gaps in service provision.

Ten guiding principles for service development

Holistic

The needs of the child with a learning disability and mental health difficulties are central to any service planning and delivery. The full range of emotional, physical, social, educational and practical needs should be considered in the context of the family, with special attention paid to parents', carers' and siblings' needs.

Child-centred planning

Service development and delivery should have the child's welfare as paramount. There should be recognition that 'children are children first', regardless of the level of their learning disability and mental health difficulties. The intention should be to develop intervention plans to meet the child's needs rather than reflect service needs. It is essential that strong links are established between children's services, child protection teams and CAMHS LD services.

Developmental framework

Throughout assessment and intervention, the difficulties presented by the child should be considered within a developmental framework. This should pay attention to both the child's chronological age and developmental level. Children with learning disabilities often show more variable developmental profiles than those without learning disabilities. For example, their verbal skills and emotional understanding may be above what might be expected given their cognitive developmental level.

Multi-agency commissioning and consideration of referrals

For care to be effective, it should be provided across health, social, educational and voluntary agencies in a comprehensive and integrated manner. Avoiding duplication of service provision and ensuring effective communication between agencies is essential in offering care which is responsive to the child's and family's needs.

Inclusion and equality of access

Children with a learning disability and their families should have equal access to the full range of services that children without learning disabilities have in respect to all areas of health, social and educational support. They should be offered appropriate support to access ordinary services where possible, and specialist alternatives where inclusion into ordinary services is not indicated.

How can services be improved for young people with learning disabilities?

Services and individual professionals should take a pro-active and problem-solving approach in addressing the needs of children and their families. They should seek to equip themselves with any necessary knowledge base or skills to meet the needs of the child. Service development and delivery should be committed to collaborative practice which empowers children, their families and advocates to overcome their difficulties and get the support they need from service providers. Children's views should be actively sought throughout the care process, and information should be provided in a child-friendly manner to enable children to be informed about their care and be able to participate in decision-making.

Co-operative information sharing and communication

Issues of consent, confidentiality and information sharing require careful consideration for children with complex inter-agency involvement. Information should be shared between service providers to meet the needs of the child, but this should be done collaboratively with children and families.

Encompassing diversity

Professionals should encompass diversity in their planning of services, and within service delivery and evaluation. Diversity relates to the child's level of disability, as well as any cultural or gender issues. Children from minority ethnic groups who have a learning disability may be more likely to face double discrimination in relation to service access.

Therapeutic and quality services

The care pathway should enable children to access the best available local service to meet their needs. Such services should be timely, of high quality and therapeutic for the child and family, and offer both comprehensive assessments and interventions.

Autism

Over the years, different diagnostic labels have been used, such as autism, autism spectrum disorder (ASD), autism spectrum condition (ASC), pervasive developmental disorder (PDD), high-functioning autism (HFA), Asperger syndrome. This reflects the different diagnostic manuals and tools used, and the different autism profiles presented by individuals. Because of recent and upcoming changes to the main diagnostic manuals, autism spectrum disorder (ASD) is now likely to become the most commonly given diagnostic term.

Autism is a lifelong developmental disability that affects how young people perceive the world and interact with others. Autistic people see, hear and feel the world differently to other people. If you are autistic, you are autistic for life; it is not an illness or disease and cannot be cured. Often people feel that being autistic is a fundamental aspect of their identity.

Autism is a spectrum condition. All autistic people share certain difficulties, but being autistic will affect them in different ways. Some autistic people also have learning disabilities, meaning they need different levels of support. All young people on the autism spectrum learn and develop. With the right sort of support, all can be helped to live a more fulfilling life of their own choosing.

What are the main characteristics of autism?

The characteristics of autism vary from one person to another, but in order for a diagnosis to be made, a person will usually be assessed as having had persistent difficulties with social communication and social interaction together with restricted and repetitive patterns of behaviours, activities or interests since early childhood, to the extent that these limit and impair everyday functioning. Autistic people have difficulties with interpreting both verbal and non-verbal language like gestures or tone of voice. Many have a very literal understanding of language, and think people always mean exactly what they say. They may find it difficult to use or understand:

- facial expressions;

- tone of voice;

- jokes and sarcasm.

The world can seem a very unpredictable and confusing place to autistic young people, who often prefer to have a daily routine so that they know what is going to happen every day. They may want to always travel the same way to and from school or college, or eat exactly the same food for breakfast. The use of rules can also be important. It may be difficult for an autistic person to take a different approach to something once they have been taught the 'right' way to do it. People on the autism spectrum may not be comfortable with the idea of change, but may be able to cope better if they can prepare for changes in advance.

Gender differences

Autism diagnosis historically shows more boys than girls diagnosed by a ratio of one to ten; however, new research shows that girls have been under-diagnosed and the real ratio may be one to three (Banaschewski et al, 2015). Girls and young women subject to socialisation pressures and role expectations have learned to be more adept at masking their autistic traits – for example, by selecting a popular girl in class and copying their behaviour. Portrayals of autism in the media have almost always been exclusively male and research studies have universally selected only male participants.

Thus, parents, teachers and clinicians tend to be less inclined to consider an autism diagnosis for young women with social and communication problems. Many of these young women go on to develop secondary mental health problems such as anxiety, depression and self-harm. The NHS estimates there are about 700,000 people on the autism spectrum in Britain based on the old gender ratio of one to ten (Doherty et al, 2016). If the new ratio was used, one to three, it would mean that 300,000 girls and young women have been omitted from the national tally.

✎ Activity 3.3

❖ Think about what kind of support can help.
❖ Can you or your agency deliver this support?

▭ Commentary

The main goals when supporting children with autism are to lessen associated deficits and family distress, and to increase quality of life and functional independence. In general, higher IQs are correlated with greater responsiveness to treatment and improved treatment outcomes. No single treatment is best and treatment is typically tailored to the child's needs. Families and the educational system are the main resources for treatment. Studies of interventions have methodological problems that prevent definitive conclusions about efficacy; however, the development of evidence-based interventions has advanced in recent years. Many psycho-social interventions have some positive evidence, suggesting that some form of treatment is preferable to no treatment. Intensive, sustained special education programmes and behaviour early in life can help children acquire self-care, social and job skills, and often improve functioning and decrease symptom severity and maladaptive behaviours. Available approaches include applied behaviour (ABA), developmental models, structured teaching, speech and language therapy, social skills therapy and occupational therapy.

The mental health needs of young offenders

According to figures published by the House of Lords Library, the amount that councils plan to spend on youth services has dropped by 53.6 per cent between 2011 and 2018 (House of Lords, 2018). Youth workers consistently warn about the impact these cuts will have on preventing crime and anti-social behaviour among young people. In June 2018 there were 883 young people imprisoned. Evidence shows that 90 per cent of these young people had a diagnosable mental health disorder, histories of child abuse and many had substance abuse problems as well as personality disorders. Young offenders are among the most socially excluded groups in society and the evidence suggests that imprisonment simply exacerbates the situation. Within two years of release, 75 per cent will have been reconvicted and 47 per cent will be back in jail. If some of these young people become homeless or end up in insecure accommodation, they are between 8 and 11 times more likely to develop mental health problems.

Young offenders are three times more likely to have a mental health problem due to childhood abuse than other young people. Yet these problems are often neglected because there are poor methods for screening and assessing mental health problems within the youth justice system. Although many aspects of the delivery of services for the mental health of children in secure settings require expertise that is no more specialist than for children in the community at large, the types of problem experienced and the approaches needed to engage and work with these children with very complex needs sometimes require highly specialist, and some relatively rare, expertise in planning and supporting effective interventions.

What can be done to improve things?

• **Developing** the awareness, competence and confidence of mental health issues among all staff working in the establishment, including both site-based and visiting colleagues.

- **Offering** training, consultation and supervision to Tier 1 staff in their work of assessing, identifying and meeting mental health needs.

- **Delivering** appropriate specialist interventions for children with moderately severe mental health problems.

- **Co-working** with CAMH colleagues in providing for children with more severe and complex problems and disorders, acting to reduce premature or delayed referral to the Tier 3 CAMHS.

- **Providing** mental health expertise to inform and support those providing advocacy, speech and language therapy, family liaison, and effective approaches with girls and with children from a minority ethnic background in liaison with other staff and agencies.

- **Working** in one or more local youth offending team (YOT), providing continuity of care for children leaving a secure setting and a regular exchange of information and ideas between staff in secure settings and those working in the community.

All professional staff working in a variety of agency settings with young offenders need to develop the capacity to undertake assessment and intervention to care for and support these young people suffering from, or at risk of developing, mental health problems. Early intervention in the lives of young people involved in anti-social behaviour can make a difference to their potential for offending behaviour.

What helps reduce youth offending?

- Engaging young people in positive activities.

- Encouraging more young people to volunteer and become involved in their communities.

- Providing better information, advice and guidance to young people.

- Providing better and more personalised intensive support for young people with serious problems or who are in trouble.

Looked after children

In 2010 fewer than 65,000 children were being looked after by their local authority; now that number has increased to more than 72,000 (Department for Education,

2018). This increase has been accompanied by a reduction in overall spending on children's services. About 60 per cent of these children had been abused or neglected with a further 10 per cent coming from 'dysfunctional families'. Abuse of this nature can lead to self-harming behaviour, severe behavioural problems and depression. Evidence confirms that the mental health needs of these children and young people are overlooked and that many have established mental health problems prior to coming into local authority care. Many of these children were in foster placements and or were in children's homes, yet foster carers and residential staff are among the least qualified and supported people left to manage sometimes extreme behaviour. Specialist CAMHS services often decline to help because of the uncertain and possibly temporary nature of the child's placement which contra-indicates successful intervention. The dilemma is that without input, placements often break down as carers cannot cope, invariably leading to more placements and further deterioration in the child's mental health.

The importance of a preventive approach with children in the public care system who are more likely to be excluded from school following emotional and behavioural difficulties cannot be overstated. Teacher training that fails to adequately prepare newly qualified staff to respond to the mental health needs of pupils is considered to be a factor in the increased use of school exclusions. A preventive approach could be helpful to teaching staff and organise collaborative work aimed at preventing difficult behaviour escalating. Unless the mental health needs of these young people are addressed as part of a strategy that effectively nurtures their inclusion in school, the risk of deterioration is high. The risk factors for looked after children are probably the most extreme of any socially excluded group; they include:

- developmental delay, school failure, communication difficulty;

- low self-esteem, parent/carer conflict, family breakdown;

- rejection, abuse, parental mental illness, alcohol/drug abuse;

- poverty, homelessness, loss.

The risk of cultural dislocation

The sense of dislocation felt by individual children and young people and their families is illustrated by noting the experience of socially excluded groups such as Roma, gypsy and travellers who may be included in recent groups of asylum and refugee-seeking families escaping ethnic 'cleansing' from the Balkan region of Central and Eastern Europe. These families have a long history of persecution and flight from discrimination. Roma, gypsy and traveller families who have for many years made their home in Britain are probably one of the most socially excluded groups of people living in Britain. Unemployment among Roma/gypsies is in the region of 70 per cent, while increasing numbers of children are failing to complete even a basic education.

These factors – particularly the lack of proper education – are risk factors for the development of psychological problems in young people. The overall context of social exclusion means an absence of contact with preventive services or the positive interaction with peers necessary for developmental attainment. Sensitive therapeutic work can help families begin the process of re-establishing patterns of behaviour that can sustain and nurture the personal growth of all concerned. Effort is required to enhance the engagement process with these families through:

• gaining an understanding of the concept of culture;

• appreciating your own culture;

• a desire to facilitate effective communication;

• an appreciation of the varying perceptions of family process across cultures;

• a desire to work with families considering their cultural values.

The experiences of children and young people uprooted by force or covert pressure can lead to a sense of loss, which is magnified by a sense of not belonging. These twin feelings can result in a kind of cultural bereavement which can get mixed up with the adolescent developmental process that requires a sense of belonging. Migration itself is a journey or transition and if the young person is simultaneously negotiating a crucial phase of transition from childhood to adulthood, problems may arise. The yearning for belonging involves being able to risk relationship and loss, whereas it is probably more useful to be able to belong to multiple worlds rather than feel excluded from them.

What does a sense of belonging mean?

This sense of belonging is enhanced by the capacity for sharing language, customs, and intersubjective experiences. A sense of sameness or identification begins to be developed in infancy when unacceptable emotions are taken in by another and the way they are returned. This secure base or containment offered by parents or staff working with them is crucial in the child developing a tolerance of difference. The importance and subtleties of understanding the meaning of what is projected, and what can be fed back, mean that we have to work hard within the reflective space when addressing issues of sameness and difference with children and adolescents.

Where adults may experience mental health problems, it is usually considered that the presence of a second parent in the home is a mitigating factor in moderating the impact on children and young people. However, this is based on Eurocentric studies that are not related to key relationships in different cultural family groupings. Research indicates that a grandparent relationship could be crucial or that access to a supportive adult outside the family home, contact with peers through school or sport, and a reliable social life all help the child or young person cope.

✏ Activity 3.4 Case illustration

The following case study examines the skills that could be used when developing a plan and reviewing its progress. As a practitioner you have inherited the case from a colleague who has moved jobs, leaving a risky situation in which the mother is finding it difficult to trust anyone.

Ms B is a depressed young Albanian Muslim woman with three children under five years of age exhibiting disturbed behaviour and a ten year old at primary school with poor attendance. The family are refugees and have experienced severe trauma in recent years. Her partner, who is ten years her senior, has been involved with drug and alcohol abuse and is suspected of abusing her. She is terrified her children will be removed because she is unable to care for them properly or protect them from the violence of her partner. Ms B is hostile to social workers, health visitors and teachers who have expressed concerns about the welfare of all four children. She feels persecuted, does not want any involvement and resents any interference in her life. The plan summary could look something like this:

- 🔍 Younger children to attend nursery daily.
- 🔍 Ms B to play with the younger children once a day.
- 🔍 Ms B to attend domestic violence survivors group.
- 🔍 Ms B to take ten year old to school.
- 🔍 Partner to attend anger management course.
- 🔍 Partner to attend drug counselling.
- 🔍 Family network to visit Ms B weekly.

💬 Commentary

While the main focus of intervention must be on the care and safety of the children, practitioners also need to engage Ms B by addressing her own needs for safety and protection. She is aware that her partner will harm her if she asks him to leave so she is stuck in an impossible dilemma. If he stays, the practitioner will allege she is failing to protect the children; if she tries to make her partner leave, she will endanger herself as well as the children. If staff acknowledge this dilemma in an uncritical way without blaming Ms B or by pretending that there is a simple solution, then they are more likely to begin the process of gaining her confidence and working collaboratively rather than coercively.

The context of her culture and religion are important factors in seeking to understand the complexities of her situation. The worker needs to be open and direct about this without giving the false impression of knowing how she feels or by signalling discomfort or embarrassment at such sensitive matters. Consideration should be given to employing an interpreter or translator even though she may be able to make herself understood, as this will signal a respectful approach and provide a cultural connection that will be emotionally supportive.

Engaging Ms B in a conversation about her experiences as a wife and mother in Albania and comparing her life with how it is now will open up a rich seam of information, which simultaneously can serve a therapeutic purpose. Getting Ms B to list her worries and concerns about the children will enable her to demonstrate that she is a capable mother and help you appreciate the emotional aspects of her experiences. Attempts to engage her partner need to be made but not at the risk of inflaming the situation or putting her and the children at greater risk.

You can then help her consider ways of tackling these worries in small, practical ways before addressing the major issue of her complex relationship with her partner. The review needs to examine every element of the plan, check whether it is happening, which agency is responsible for what element, what impact the intervention is having on each child's mental health and whether additional needs have emerged or alternative interventions need to be considered. The review should check whether the plan is addressing and meeting each individual child's developmental needs, mental health and emotional well-being, as well as their collective needs as a sibling group.

It also needs to examine the parenting capacity of Ms B on her own and conjointly with her partner. The wider family context should be explored to see what pattern of relationships exists with a view to encouraging increased supportive contact. If no immediate family exist then a wider definition of 'family' could identify religious, spiritual or social support networks. In a safer environment, the children's mental health may regress and deteriorate so it is important to distinguish these temporary healing experiences from sustained developmental problems due to continued abuse.

Ms B may not be able to manage every aspect of the plan because it feels overwhelming. For example, the survivors group may be poorly organised by unskilled people who cannot meet her particular needs. She may be the only Muslim and the target of racist abuse within the group. Thought needs to be given to finding the right group for her particular needs rather than just the first available resource. However, she may be succeeding in getting the older child to school and she must be genuinely congratulated for this.

By establishing a solid platform for her to feel supported, empowered and capable of defining her children's needs, she will be more likely to feel strong enough to deal with her violent partner. If the situation became more risky then the practitioner would need to confront Ms B with the likely consequences of inaction on her part. However, this needs to be done alongside offering maximum support by all agencies involved in a co-ordinated package. Effective review and closure will more likely happen if a collaborative relationship with Ms B has developed which will enable her to seek further help in the future if required.

What are the elements of socially inclusive practice?

Workers have to assess needs, evaluate risks and allocate resources in a way that is equitable as far as possible for a wide range of young people in various situations. Challenging oppression in relation to key issues such as poverty and social marginalisation that underpin interactions in social welfare requires a holistic approach to change that tackles oppression at the personal, institutional and cultural levels. An empowering practice can contribute to the defence of marginalised people using an overarching progressive framework.

✏ Activity 3.5

✎ Review the chapter up to this point and then note down some of the core elements that in your mind constitute a socially inclusive practice.
✎ Now compare your notes with the following material.

⬚ Commentary

A review of the elements that constitute a socially inclusive practice lists four core intervention skills necessary to build on an authentic and integrated practice that reflects humanitarian values. These elements have much in common with counselling and therapeutic approaches.

• **Social entrepreneurship:** the ability to initiate, lead and carry through problem-solving strategies in collaboration with other people in all kinds of social networks.

- **Reflection:** the worker's ability to pattern or make sense of information, in whatever form, including the impact of their own behaviour and that of the organisation on others.

- **Challenging:** refers to your ability to confront people effectively with their responsibilities, their problem-perpetuating/creating behaviours and their conflicting interests.

- **Reframing:** the ability to help redefine circumstances in ways which lead towards problem resolution.

However, if we wish to promote the conditions for change within a young person suffering from mental health problems we need to attend to the constraints outside the person. We must counteract oppression, mobilise users' rights and promote choice, yet have to act within organisational and legal structures which users experience as oppressive. Finding your way through this dilemma and reaching compromises, or discovering the potential for creative thinking and practice, are the challenges and opportunities open to staff committed to a socially inclusive practice. This means treating people as a whole, and as being in interaction with their environment, of respecting their understanding and interpretation of their experience, and seeing clients at the centre of what workers are doing. A psycho-social perspective offers a vast reservoir of knowledge and skills to bring to bear on the multiple problems of socially excluded young people and their mental well-being.

How to develop anti-racist and anti-oppressive practice

Anti-racist and anti-oppressive practice are repeatedly referred to in the literature and have a long historical lineage as part of the social justice basis of modern health and social care practice. The concepts are backed up in counselling and psychotherapy codes of conduct, ethical guidance and occupational standards defined by central and local government requiring services to meet the needs of diverse cultures and combat discrimination. They are part and parcel of what attracts many of us into helping work in the first place. Translating good intentions into daily practice is however harder than it might at first appear.

For example, in the case of childcare practice there is still a tendency for social workers to proceed with assessment on the basis that the mother is the main responsible carer with the father taking a minor role. Women are perceived therefore as responsible for any problems with their child or children and for their protection. You may feel that this reflects the reality, especially in cases of single parenthood, or domestic violence where fathers are absent or a threat. Anti-oppressive practice requires in these situations acknowledgement of the mother's predicament and multiple dilemmas. It requires an informed culturally competent practice using feminist and psycho-social theory to evaluate the situation and seek every small opportunity to support the mother and engage the father. The combination of personal guilt felt by women in these circumstances, with a mother-blaming tendency in society, can erode their precarious coping skills and paradoxically increase risk factors for child and adolescent mental health problems.

In this context, it is important to consider the specific challenges faced by South Asian adolescent girls as members of immigrant families. A study of Indian, Pakistani and Bangladeshi families in Montreal, Canada found that gender roles prevalent within each culture were maintained through segregation, control over social activities and arranged marriage (Walker, 2016). The adolescents felt that their parents and communities have more stringent rules for female socialisation than any other community. Because of the high levels of connectedness in the nature of family relationships, these adolescent girls perceived a high social cost attached to protest or dissent in relation to the cultural rules resulting in elevated levels of stress.

A history of childhood mental health problems is strongly indicated in the risk factors for developing adult mental health problems. Adult black people are over-represented in mental health services. It is imperative therefore that the needs of all black and ethnic minority children vulnerable to mental health problems are addressed early and competently in order to prevent later problems. Your anti-racist work in multi-disciplinary ways as part of inter-agency groups co-ordinating efforts to support the child and family through temporary or moderate difficulties could be critical. As a worker using culturally competent skills, you can support other staff in statutory or voluntary resources by offering a more holistic evaluation and assessment of the family process adapted to take account of cultural diversity.

✎ Activity 3.6

🔪 Discuss with a colleague how you might change your practice to show that you were making an effort to understand how different families made sense of child and adolescent mental health problems.

🔪 Consider the community you are part of and whether your agency is doing everything it can to reach all families within it and enhance social inclusion.

⌨ Commentary

One way of demonstrating this is to exclude the risk of misinterpretation or underplaying significant emotional and behavioural characteristics in socially excluded

Chapter 3: Why are diversity, cultural awareness and social inclusion important?

69

families. An understanding of the reluctance and resistance of black parents to consider a mental health explanation for their child's behaviour or emotional state is important when considering how to engage parents or carers from diverse cultural backgrounds in the process of support. It is equally important to make efforts to understand cultural explanations and belief systems around disturbed behaviour as part of risk assessment work. Respecting rather than challenging difference should be the starting point for finding ways of moving forward in partnership and co-operation. The dilemma in aspiring to practice in socially inclusive ways is in balancing this respect with knowledge and evidence of the consequences of untreated emerging mental health problems.

The characteristics of non-Western societies such as collectivism, community and physical explanations for emotional problems are in contrast to Western concepts of individualism and psychological explanations. The Western model of mental illness ignores the religious or spiritual aspects of the culture in which it is based. However, Eastern, African and Native American cultures tend to integrate them. Spirituality and religion can be critical components of a family's well-being, offering a source of strength and hope in trying circumstances. You need to address this dimension as part of the constellation of factors affecting black children and adolescents, avoiding stereotyping, and bearing in mind the positive and sometimes negative impact spiritual or religious beliefs might have on their mental health.

Basing your practice on socially inclusive principles is about how you define yourself as a worker and your relationship to service users. You cannot bolt-on a bit of anti-oppressive practice; it has to be part and parcel of all your everyday practice as a contribution to tackling poverty, social justice, and the structural causes of inequality. This goes against practice guidance that advocates a maintenance or care management role for practitioners and might bring you into conflict with managers and local politicians who have a narrow focus. Wherever you position yourself, you will probably find yourself occupying different roles at different times in your work regardless of your explicit intentions. This is because if you are client-centred then you will engage with young people in partnership informed by psycho-social practice to help meet their needs in order to maintain them in their current circumstances, or support them in their struggle towards social inclusion.

⚒ Summary of key points

✦ No worker can be effective without combining the individual psychology of the child or adolescent with the social context of their problems to gain a holistic picture. Similarly, no therapeutic work can properly work with a child and family's internal problems in the absence of the wider context of their experience of social exclusion.

✦ The evidence confirms that the gap between rich and poor is widening, there are more children living in poverty, the prison population is at its highest recorded level, and disabled people are more likely to live in poverty or be unemployed than non-disabled people. Children from working-class families are less likely to receive a further or higher education and black families are more likely to live in poor housing.

✦ In a postcolonial world, the rights and expectations of Indigenous people to reparation and how they are perceived are important issues in the context of achieving culturally competent practice. The disparities between developed and developing economies under the influence of globalisation are becoming more pronounced, incorporating new forms of cultural domination.

✦ A socially inclusive practice can be helpful when addressing issues of loss and bereavement with ethnic minority families where earlier generations were split up during periods of economic growth. Refugee and asylum-seeking children are among the most disadvantaged ethnic minority group for whom socially inclusive practice is essential. Some are unaccompanied, and many affected by extreme circumstances might include those witnessing murder of parents or kin, dislocation from school and community, and severing of important friendships. Lack of extended family support, loss of home and prolonged insecurity add to their sense of vulnerability. These experiences can trigger symptoms of post-traumatic stress disorder and a variety of mental health problems.

✦ The characteristics of non-Western societies such as collectivism, community and physical explanations for emotional problems are in contrast to Western concepts of individualism and psychological explanations. An understanding of the resistance of some parents to consider a mental health explanation for their child's behaviour or emotional state is important when balancing the knowledge and evidence of the consequences of untreated emerging mental health problems.

Further reading

Bernard, S and Turk, J (2009) *Developing Mental Health Services for Children and Adolescents with Learning Disabilities: A Toolkit for Clinicians*. London: RCP.

Campbell, S, Morley, D and Catchpole, R (2016) *Critical Issues in Child and Adolescent Mental Health*. London: Palgrave Macmillan.

Dwivedi, K N (2002) *Meeting the Needs of Ethnic Minority Children*. London: Jessica Kingsley.

Malek, M and Joughin, C (2004) *Mental Health Services for Minority Ethnic Children and Adolescents*. London: Jessica Kingsley.

Robinson, L (2013) Racism and Mental Health. In Walker, S (ed) *Modern Mental Health: Critical Perspectives on Psychiatric Practice* (pp 118–28). St Albans: Critical Publishing.

Walker, S (2005) *Culturally Competent Therapy with Children and Young People*. London: Palgrave Macmillan.

Internet resources

Black, Asian and Minority Ethnic Young People: **www.bameednetwork.com**

Muslim Youth Helpline: **www.myh.org.uk**

Children's Society: **www.childrenssociety.org.uk**

Chapter 4: How to provide support and intervention

Introduction

Every intervention should have a purpose and, as much as possible, that purpose should be identified clearly and openly as part of the agreement established with children, families and other key individuals and professionals involved. The seemingly routine task of an assessment interview can be thought of as an intervention in its own right because of the opportunity to gain a greater understanding of young people and their situations in a therapeutic way. That is, by using the opportunity to establish a helping relationship as the basis for initiating change, rather than seeing it as an administrative task.

The choice of intervention open to workers in child mental health work is necessarily broad because of the wide variety of psychological and social factors influencing the child or young person being helped. The literature itself offers a sometimes bewildering array of methods and models of intervention, apart from the wider psychiatric, psychological and therapeutic texts available to guide the helping process with individuals, families or groups. Public health, education, social and fiscal policy interventions by local and central government agencies also impact on children's welfare generally and need to be taken into account.

Before embarking on any one form of intervention though, you need to reflect on the ethical questions raised by the choices made and the potential consequences. The legal contexts for intervening in children and young people's lives are considered in Chapter 7 and are relevant to this discussion because of the link with consent and competence to understand the choices offered. For example, individual counselling or therapy may succeed in helping a young person to develop a sense of self, but in so doing the experience may alienate them from their family. Family therapy may result in the improvement of a child with emotional difficulties, but in the process of the work siblings may be adversely affected or the parental marriage/partnership exposed as problematic. Even though you may not deliver the work yourself, the act of referring to a specialist resource offering specific help means you are sanctioning a potentially powerful intervention in the lives of the child and their family.

✎ Activity 4.1

What are the dilemmas in deciding how to help?

💬 Commentary

A worker who feels that a child is bottling up their feelings and needs to learn to express them in counselling may be causing additional stress to the child who is expected, within their community or cultural context, to be developing self-control and containment of emotions. A young person who is displaying destructive obsessional behaviour as a means of managing their stress may be given a behavioural or psychodynamic intervention by a worker, depending on the particular preference of that individual worker. However, each intervention comes with its own set of assumptions and potential consequences in terms of generating other stressors. The same intervention could be given to two children with the same problem, but only one of them might benefit. These ethical dilemmas are important to acknowledge and reflect upon before proceeding with any course of action. The crucial point is to ensure the most effective intervention is offered for the appropriate problem with the right child.

Why is early intervention important?

The principle of preparing people for potential difficulties is useful and resonates with pro-active initiatives in schools, youth clubs and resources such as telephone helplines/ internet discussion groups and campaigns, to reach out to children and young people before they reach a crisis. Linking specific therapeutic interventions with agreed outcomes is problematic due to the network of variables potentially impacting on a child or young person's development. It is notoriously difficult to accurately predict the effect of specific interventions, especially when there is a lack of a research and evaluation culture in an agency (Walker, 2011). Equally, it is even harder to measure the impact of preventive or early intervention programmes because of the impossibility of proving that something did not happen.

Children and adolescents acquire different at-risk labels such as looked after, excluded, or young offender, affecting the variety of perceptions of their needs from the care system, education system or youth justice system. This can have a detrimental effect on efforts to plan holistically and build a coalition among different professional staff to intervene preventively. Each professional system has its own language and methodology with which to describe the same child, sometimes resulting in friction between agencies and misconceptions about how to work together and integrate interventions. Arguments over the *real* nature of a child's behaviour or the *correct* theoretical interpretation are a wasteful extravagance. In this climate the mental health needs of such children can be neglected and the opportunity for thoughtful, preventive work missed.

As well as understanding why some children develop mental health problems, it is crucially important to learn more about those who in similar circumstances do not.

Research is required to analyse the nature of these resilient children to understand whether coping strategies or skills can be transferred to other children. Positive factors such as reduced social isolation, good schooling and supportive adults outside the family appear to help. These are the very factors missing in socially excluded families who generally live in deprived conditions and suffer more socio-economic disadvantages than other children. Yet many of these children will not develop mental health problems.

Preventive practice

One of the most important preventive approaches is helping children and young people cope with the stresses they face in modern society. Every generation has to negotiate the manifestations of stress in their wider culture; therefore, relying on methods used by former generations is not useful. This is challenging to practitioners who will naturally draw from their own experiences as an instinctive resource or look for emotional resources within the young person's family. Therefore, a useful starting point is first to understand the different levels of stress experienced by children and young people.

Stress is a broad concept and includes a diverse range of experiences. It is a word that has crept into common usage to cover a wide variety of situations such as the pace of life, homework/exams, friendship rows through to the death of a grandparent, moving house/school or important relationship endings. The key is to ensure that the child themselves can categorise the level of stress. For example, whether a bereavement is an acute or moderate stress, or whether parental separation/divorce is a severe and longer-lasting stress. What helps is enabling the child or adolescent to focus on what can be done to improve the situation rather than concentrating on negative feelings. The benefits for preventive work in the area of child and adolescent mental health are likely to be positive. Reducing the likelihood of mental health problems reduces the likelihood of abuse from the parent/carer's inability to cope. Neighbourhood and community projects designed to deter anti-social behaviour and channel youth energies into purposeful activity all have their role to play in CAMHS.

What is empowering practice?

Services geared towards the needs of specific age groups of children or young people, or adults, can determine the type of help offered and whether it is perceived as family or individual support. While age is one factor, the type of problem, its degree and duration will also determine where and how help might be offered. Practitioners working in an empowering or participatory way will strive to find, or offer themselves as, the most acceptable and accessible type of intervention resource. However, dilemmas will present themselves when some parents and/or children and young people express rigid views about what they want against the best available evidence of what can help.

For example, a parent might insist on a child receiving individual counselling to quell troublesome behaviour, whereas all the evidence points towards couple/marital counselling. Your offer of help may be rejected because parents insist on a consultation with a psychologist or psychiatrist, even though this may reinforce their beliefs that their child is the one with the problem. This may inhibit engaging with them in a partnership approach designed to widen their field of vision from scapegoating a child who may be simply displaying the symptoms of familial/marital or environmental causes. These beliefs and perceptions are rooted in a number of factors such as professional status/wanting the best for their child, but they are also driven by deep feelings of guilt, anxiety, fear and anger. Using an empowering model will enable you to respectfully address these in congruent, empathic, unconditional positive ways. Practice based on an empowering model:

- concentrates on the present rather than the past;

- attempts to help people achieve equilibrium between their inner emotional states and the pressures they face in the outside world;

- uses the child or parent's relationship with the practitioner actively.

Reflective practice

Reflective practice is considered to be the hallmark of modern practice among professionals working with people in a helping role. It has resonance with the ideas contained in psycho-social skills of practitioner self-awareness and the feelings generated in the helping relationship between the worker and client. It is recommended as a way of evaluating the impact of intervention and done in partnership can be empowering for some clients. Supervision or professional consultation in the area of child and adolescent mental health is a crucial component of reflective practice. A manager with the skills to offer case consultation combined with management supervision is ideal but probably a rarity.

Practitioners involved with families or in situations where child mental health problems are an issue require quality consultation separate from the administrative and managerial aspects of their work. A senior colleague or other professional might be the best resource as long as they can help you disentangle your own feelings from those being generated during potentially emotionally intense work. Simple concepts such as transference and projection used in a pragmatic way can go a long way towards increasing effectiveness and clarity in confusing and worrying situations.

Analysing and planning

In developing a deeper understanding of a young person's difficulties with a view to deciding on intervention, you can draw on a range of theories and methods. Differing hypotheses result from viewing situations with the aid of these theories. This is healthy although it can be unhelpful if it leads to confusion and drift in your practice. At its best it can help guard against the temptation to claim a single truth in any situation. Forming alternative understandings and explanations is a good habit to acquire. However, judgements have to be made and will be demanded by managers and expected in legal proceedings where they will be examined and tested. The most desirable practice is where an interpretation is helpful to both you and your client in contributing to holistic planning, developing solutions, and where it is rooted in values of respect and anti-oppressive practice.

Maintaining a reflexive stance helps you consider the consequences of using particular theories and encouraging clients to develop their own theories about their situations. You will need more than one model of assessment and intervention to enable you to meet the needs of all your clients – if not, you will be like a plumber with only one spanner. Having a grasp of different models of practice should enable you, together with the client, to select the most appropriate model, and help you maintain a degree of open-mindedness. This process will enable you to plan your intervention by integrating and analysing information and forming a judgement in partnership with your client in a multi-disciplinary context. Table 4.1 offers a schematic representation of how to ensure that a plan is organised, structured and incorporates everyone necessary.

✒ Activity 4.2

🔨 Consider how to collate important information about a young person you are starting to work with.

🔨 What are the key elements to incorporate in planning support?

💬 Commentary

Integrating knowledge, skills and values in analysing information and being able to weigh its significance and priority as a basis for effective planning is a demanding task. Sound planning will happen provided the following elements in the decision-making process are delineated:

Table 4.1 Areas for consideration when planning multi-disciplinary care

Initial discussion	Identify core group staff	Collate contributions to plan	Specify meeting dates	Clarify responsibility boundaries	Clarify assessment depth
The core group	Purpose and function	Methods to promote participatory practice	Anticipate potential inter-agency problems	Agree protocols for more attendees	Management of meeting: minutes/ feedback
The plan	Overall aim	Timescale to implement	Methods to engage child and family	Agree procedures for changes to plan	Evaluation and plan monitoring
The key worker	Co-ordination	Direct work with child or family	Keeping an overview	Clarify joint working tasks	Manage inter-agency problems
The review	The remit of the review	Delegation of core group decisions	Guidance on reporting to the review	Enabling contributions from child and family	Providing support to staff

- **Being critically aware of and taking into account the decision-making contexts:** knowledge of legal requirements and agency procedures are critical ingredients of planning what is possible and permissible. Statutory duty has to be balanced against your endeavour to take a holistic perspective of the situation.

- **Involving the client to the highest feasible level:** there can be four levels – being told; being consulted; being a partner; and being in control. A key skill is to fit the level of involvement to the nature of the particular planning situation.

- **Consulting with all stakeholders:** there could be numerous stakeholders involved in your work with a particular young person. Some will have more systematic contact but only general knowledge about the client, but they could be just as valuable as someone with limited contact but who has specialised knowledge. A range of perceptions can either enhance the clarity in a situation or confirm your hypothesis, or produce a disparate and confusing picture, which hinders rather than helps.

- **Being clear in your thinking and aware of your emotions:** a heightened element of self-awareness is always useful. Over-reacting to a situation on the basis of tiredness, stress and the day of the week or simply false information needs to be guarded against. Equally, under-reacting to a risky situation because of feelings of pity, empathy or over-optimism can contribute to an escalation of risk factors.

- **Producing a well-reasoned frame of the decision situation that is consistent with the available information:** through framing processes you can shape the information into a picture of the situation, planning goals and a set of options. Listing key factors and considering the weight to give to each requires knowledge, experience and the capacity for short- and long-term predictions of the consequences of various interventions.

- **Basing your course of action on a systematic appraisal of the options:** the plan could be based on the principle that a statutory duty overrides the traumatic impact of the subsequent intervention, or on which option is likely to provide the best outcome in the context of risk assessment and available supportive resources.

What skills and strategies are required for integrated intervention?

Holistic planning and intervention requires you to draw upon a number of skills and strategies. One of the most fundamental is previous learning often referred to as *practice wisdom*. Learning arises as a result of the four-stage process of concrete experience; reflective observation; abstract conceptualisation; and active experimentation. You can use this model to describe and facilitate the application of your knowledge and theory to assessment and planning practice. The following points can guide you in this process.

- Guard against the false belief in theoryless practice.

- Research-minded practice can help integrate theory and practice.

- The critical incident technique is a way of analysing a situation where strong emotions were raised in your practice and which interfered with your ability to function effectively then or could in the future.

- Developing a group approach for narrowing the gap between theory and practice can be very effective.

- Planning intervention in your work and the decision-making process includes thinking and feeling about the situation being addressed.

The key skills in direct work

Table 4.2 details the recommended treatments and support strategies for children and adolescents suffering mental health problems. They have been collated on the basis of considerable research (Rutter et al, 2008) into effectiveness but from an evidence base that is not yet methodologically robust. Studies examining their efficacy tend to be done by doctors in clinical settings under controlled conditions. They do not therefore match with the practice reality for staff in non-specialist contexts undertaking several different roles. However, they serve a very useful purpose in providing knowledge and information about how mental health problems can be tackled. Many interventions and the theoretical base informing them are the same across a number of professional groups. Research by Rutter et al (2008) also confirms that core interpersonal skills transcend disparate treatments, methods and models.

Table 4.2 Recommended treatments for children and young people's mental health disorders

DEPRESSION
For mild depression: 'watchful waiting' for up to four weeks. Non-directive therapy, group cognitive behavioural therapy (CBT) or guided self-help may be beneficial.
Moderate to severe depression: psychological therapy as a first-line treatment (eg individual CBT, interpersonal therapy or shorter-term family therapy) for at least three months.
Antidepressant medication (selective serotonin reuptake inhibitors or SSRIs) may be considered, particularly for adolescents, but only in combination with psychological therapy and if there is no response to psychological therapy after four to six sessions.
Family therapy or individual child psychotherapy if the child or young person is still not responsive may be considered. Advice on exercise, sleep and nutrition may also help.

ANXIETY AND PHOBIAS INCLUDING OBSESSIVE COMPULSIVE DISORDER (OCD) AND BODY DYSMORPHIC DISORDER (BDD)
Behavioural therapies and CBT, sometimes involving family or carers (particularly if the child is under 11 or there is high parental anxiety), or exposure and response prevention (for young people with OCD or BDD who have not responded to guided self-help). However, CBT only appears to be effective in 50 per cent of cases treated in randomised controlled trials.
Antidepressant medication (SSRIs), usually in combination with a psychological therapy, may be used for social anxieties, OCD or BDD that have not responded to CBT. The provision of information, advice and support at school may also be helpful.

POST-TRAUMATIC STRESS DISORDER (PTSD)
Trauma-focused CBT, adapted to suit the child or young person's age, circumstances and level of development.
Eye movement desensitisation and reprocessing (EMDR) is used but there has been limited research into this to date. EMDR involves focusing on a particular physical action while thinking about the traumatic experiences in order to change the individual's thoughts and feelings about those experiences.

CONDUCT DISORDERS INCLUDING OPPOSITIONAL DEFIANT DISORDER (ODD)

Group parent-training programmes led by a therapist, particularly for less severe conduct problems. On average, two-thirds of children under ten years whose parents take part show improvement, with effects detectable for up to four years.

Parent training for conduct disorders in adolescents seems to have limited effectiveness.

Problem-solving and social skills training may be helpful if used in combination with parent training for 8 to 12 year olds, or where problems are more severe. However, the benefits may be short term.

Family therapy for adolescents and young people with moderate conduct problems, combined with CBT where appropriate.

Multisystemic therapy (MST) is an intensive programme that involves a therapist working with a family in their home to help them change their behaviour patterns, resolve conflicts, introduce rules that will improve the conduct of their child, and reduce opportunities for delinquent behaviour. It is probably the most effective treatment for adolescents with severe and enduring problems.

Therapeutic foster care with trained and experienced foster parents can help children and young people with severe and enduring problems.

Medication may help in particular cases, after other forms of treatment have been tried and where conduct disorders are associated with hyperactivity.

ATTENTION DEFICIT HYPERACTIVITY DISORDER (ADHD)

Parent-training programmes (developed for the management of children with conduct disorders) as the first-line treatment for pre-school children. It should also be offered to the parents of school-age children and young people with moderate ADHD. Parent training/ education can improve a child or young person's compliance, boost parental self-esteem and reduce parental stress, although it is not effective in all cases. It may also be used in combination with a group or individual treatment programme (such as CBT or social skills training) for the child or young person.

Stimulant medication is the first-line treatment for school-age children and young people with severe ADHD. Research shows it can reduce hyperactivity and improve concentration in 75 per cent of treated children. However, it may lead to mild growth suppression, particularly when used for continuous treatment, so breaks are advisable. It should always form part of a comprehensive treatment plan that includes psychological, behavioural and educational advice and therapy.

Changes to diet and nutrition (for example, avoiding foods that contain high levels of sugar and artificial colourings, and carbonated drinks) may help some children and young people. ADHD has been linked to deficiencies in essential fatty acids, and there is evidence that taking Omega-3 and Omega-6 fatty acids has a positive effect on reading and spelling and ADHD-related behaviours.

Exposure and Response Prevention (ERP) works on the principle that if you stay in a stressful situation long enough, you become used to it and your anxiety decreases – ie you gradually face the situation you fear (exposure) but stop yourself from doing your usual compulsive rituals (response prevention) and wait for your anxiety to pass.

SCHIZOPHRENIA

Medication (eg anti-psychotic medicines called 'atypical neuroleptics') is the primary form of treatment.

Specialist care (eg support from crisis-resolution and home-treatment teams).

Psychological therapies, particularly CBT and family therapy (these have been found to benefit adults with psychosis but less is known about how much they help younger people).

BIPOLAR DISORDER

Medication (eg lithium, neuroleptics or mood stabilisers) is the primary form of treatment.

Psychological therapies may also be used as part of treatment, eg to manage depressive symptoms.

EATING DISORDERS

Anorexia nervosa:

Psychological therapies (such as CBT, cognitive analytic therapy [CAT], interpersonal psychotherapy, psychodynamic psychotherapy).

Family therapy focused specifically on eating disorders.

In-patient care as necessary, including psychological or behaviour therapy that focuses on eating behaviour, attitudes to weight and shape, and wider issues.

Bulimia nervosa:

Self-help in the first instance.

Antidepressant drugs may also be offered as an alternative or additional first step.

Family therapy

CBT for bulimia (CBT-BN), adapted to suit the patient's age, circumstances and level of development, and involving their family as appropriate.

Interpersonal psychotherapy or other psychological treatments may be considered as an alternative, but further research is needed into their effectiveness.

Behaviour therapy may also be used with children and young people who are being treated in hospital to help them put on weight. Treatment must involve the management of physical aspects of the condition as the risk of morbidity is high.

DELIBERATE SELF-HARM

Specific advice on self-management of superficial injuries, harm-minimisation techniques and alternative coping strategies for people who repeatedly self-injure. Helping young people to distract themselves from self-harm by using a red water-soluble felt tip pen to mark their skin, rather than cutting themselves.

Developmental group psychotherapy with other young people who have repeatedly self-harmed may be effective in reducing repetition.

Family therapy may help in addressing the issues that cause self-harm.

> **SUBSTANCE ABUSE**
>
> **Family therapy and MST** may be effective in reducing substance abuse and tackling related problems.
>
> **Motivational interviewing** is a form of counselling in which the counsellor discusses with the child or young person the advantages and disadvantages of changing his or her behaviour. This may be effective, and also preventive programmes in schools can be run that build personal, social and resistance skills.

Methods and models of support

The following methods and models of practice are not an exclusive list. Within each are specific skill sets informed by sound theory and research (Rutter et al, 2008). They have been chosen from the range of modern methods and models available to aid clarity in selection of the most appropriate components of an effective intervention in child and adolescent mental health work. Discussion of the merits of defining methods and models of practice, and examination of the distinctions between terms such as practice approach, orientation and perspective, has been avoided for the sake of brevity and to avoid adding to the confusion already highlighted in the literature.

Systemic practice

Employing a systemic or systems model in child and adolescent mental health practice is characterised by the key notion that individual children and young people have a social context which influences, to a greater or lesser extent, their behaviour and their perception of their problem. This way of working is embedded in modern CAMHS practice. An important social context is that of the family and this has led to the practice of family therapy as a method of practice. It offers a broad framework for intervention, enabling the mapping all of the important elements affecting families as well as a method of working with those elements to effect beneficial change. Key features include:

• convening family meetings to give a voice to everyone connected to an individual's problem (eg family group conference);

• constructing a genogram (family tree) with a family to help identify the quality of relationships;

• harnessing the strengths of families to support the young person;

- using a problem-oriented style to energise the family to find their own solutions;

- assisting in the development of insight into patterns of behaviour and communication within the family system;

- adopting a neutral position as far as possible in order to avoid accusations of bias/collusion.

Many professionals use this model as an overarching framework to help guide their practice. It is particularly useful to use to clarify situations where there is multi-agency and multi-professional involvement in clients' lives. It can help the drawing of boundaries and sort out who does what in often complex, fast-moving and confusing situations. It also helps avoid the assumption that the individual child or young person should necessarily be the main focus for intervention.

Psychodynamic practice

The model offers a concept of the mind, its mechanisms and a method of understanding why some children behave in seemingly repetitive, destructive ways. It is the essential one-to-one helping relationship involving advanced listening and communication skills. The model provides a framework to address profound disturbances and inner conflicts within children and adolescents around issues of loss, attachment, anxiety and personal development. Key ideas such as defence mechanisms, and transference in the relationship between the worker and client, can be extremely helpful in reviewing the work being undertaken, and in the process of supervision. The model helps evaluate the strong feelings aroused in particular work situations, where for example a client transfers feelings and attitudes onto the worker that derive from an earlier significant relationship. Counter-transference occurs when you try to live up to that expectation and behave, for example, like the client's parent. Key features include the following points.

- It is a useful way of attempting to understand seemingly irrational behaviour.

- The notion of defence mechanisms is a helpful way of assessing male adolescents who have difficulty expressing their emotions.

- It acknowledges the influence of past events/attachments and can create a healthy suspicion about surface behaviour.

- The development of insight can be a particularly empowering experience to enable children and young people to understand themselves and take more control over their own lives.

- The model has influenced a listening, accepting approach that avoids over-directiveness.

- It can be used to assess which developmental stage is reflected in the child or young person's behaviour and to gauge the level of anxiety/depression.

Cognitive behavioural practice

Practice with this model is based on the key concept that all behaviour is learned and therefore available to be unlearned or changed. It offers a framework for assessing the pattern of behaviour in children and adolescents and a method for altering their thinking, feeling and behaviour. The intervention can be used with individuals and groups of young people. It aims to help them become aware of themselves, link thoughts and emotions, and enable them to acquire new life skills. Using this approach, you would decide on the goals/new behaviours to be achieved with the client, those that are clear but also capable of measurement. The four major behavioural techniques include desensitisation, aversion therapy, operant conditioning and modelling. Key features include:

- using the ABC formula – what are the Antecedents, the Behaviour and the Consequences of the problem;

- focusing on what behaviours are desired and reinforcing them;

- modelling and rehearsing desired behavioural patterns;

- combining behavioural and cognitive approaches to produce better results;

- gradually desensitising a child or young person to a threat or phobia.

Behavioural approaches have appeal for staff undertaking intervention because it offers a systematic, scientific approach from which to structure their practice. The approach goes some way towards encouraging participatory practice, discouraging labelling, and maintains the client's story as central. The idea of learned helplessness has the potential to bridge the gap between psychological and sociological explanations of behaviour, maintaining the focus on both social and individual factors.

Task-centred practice

Task-centred work is often cited as the most popular base for contemporary assessment and intervention practice, but it may be that it is used as a set of activities rather than as a theoretically based approach from which a set of activities flows. Key features include the following points.

- It is based on client agreement or service user acceptance of a legal justification for action.

- It aims to move from problem to goal, from what is wrong to what is needed.

- It is based around tasks which are central to the process of change and which aim to build on individual service user strengths as far as possible.

- The approach is time-limited, preserving client self-esteem and independence as far as possible.

- It is a highly structured model of practice using a building block approach so that each task can be agreed and success or not measured by moving from problem to goal.

It can serve as a basic approach for the majority of children and young people. In this approach, the problem is always the problem as defined by the client. It therefore respects their values, beliefs and perceptions. This approach encourages children and young people to select the problem they want to work on and engages them in task selection and review. It lends itself to a collaborative and empowering approach by enabling you to carry out your share of tasks and review them alongside those of the client. Time limits and task reviews aid motivation and promote optimism.

Narrative therapeutic practice

Narrative therapeutic ideas have developed in recent years among workers captivated by the notion of storytelling as a means to engage children and young people. Narrative therapeutic ideas recognise the ability children and young people have to ascribe meaning to events that serve to explain but also to influence choices about the possible courses of action. This capacity to generate and evolve new narratives and stories to make sense of experiences involves the use of culturally shared myths, legends and fairy stories. Thus, therapy is seen as not just offering new perceptions and insights but in the very nature of the conversation taking place. Narrative therapists suggest that problems are derived and maintained from the *internalisation* of oppressive ways of perceiving the self. These notions can be reinforced by parents who constantly criticise a child or who only respond negatively to behaviours. Key characteristics include the following points.

- It includes the technique of *externalising* the problem whereby the social worker encourages the child to objectify or personify the problem outside of themselves.

- The child can separate themselves from the problem instead of being seen and related to by others as *the problem*.

- Engage the child or young person in a process of exploring and resisting the problem as an unwanted impediment rather than as an integral part of their psychic constitution.

- Enable a troubled young person to begin the process of challenging self-defeating and overwhelming self-concepts.

Advantages

Children and young people who are suffering from psychological distress requiring therapeutic help may be either too young or too old to engage in cognitive and verbal communication about their feelings and experiences. The young ones may be more at ease with activities and play materials to aid expression while the older teenagers will often be difficult to engage and open up having learned the basic defence of silence. But they will all know something of fairy tales, myths and legends. Every culture has them and they are usually told during early childhood in a verbal parental or carer ritual as old as time. Earliest school literature incorporates these stories in the education curriculum precisely because they are familiar and accessible.

As part of the healing process, literature is an often *underrated* asset. Yet it carries information about families, emotions, morality, relationships and so much else in a way that can enable very damaged children to use devices such as fairy stories to help understand themselves at a deeper level. Fairy stories have the capacity to capture the child's imagination because they usually involve fantastical creatures, transformational experiences or complex predicaments in which the child can immerse themselves and relate to their inner world.

✐ Activity 4.3

🔧 Consider the above examples of support for young people with mental health problems.

🔧 Which ones are you using and which would you like to incorporate in your work?

How can mindfulness be used to help troubled young people?

Mindfulness is the psychological process of bringing one's attention to experiences occurring in the present moment, which can be developed through the practice of meditation and other training. The term *mindfulness* is a translation of the Pali term *sati*, which is a significant element of Buddhist traditions. In Buddhist teachings, mindfulness is utilised to develop self-knowledge and wisdom that gradually lead to what is described as enlightenment or the complete freedom from suffering. The recent popularity of mindfulness in the West is being used in schools and other contexts to help young people with mental health problems or those at risk of developing them.

Large population-based research studies (Campbell et al, 2016) have indicated that the practice of mindfulness is strongly correlated with greater well-being and perceived health. Studies have also shown that rumination and worry contribute to mental illnesses such as depression and anxiety, and that mindfulness-based interventions are effective in the reduction of both rumination and worry. A number of therapeutic applications based on mindfulness for helping people who are experiencing a variety of psychological conditions is being employed to reduce depression, stress and anxiety. The practice of mindfulness also appears to be a preventive strategy to halt the development of mental health problems. Over 5,000 teachers in the UK have been trained to teach mindfulness, according to the Mindfulness Initiative (2019), and that number is growing all the time.

Classroom or group-based mindfulness exercise

An effective method to introduce mindfulness and meditation into your group or classroom is to engage in a mindfulness of the body: relaxation exercise. This exercise not only helps to improve a young person's mindfulness but functions to relax the tension and tightness that has built up within the body and mind. The following is a step-by-step script of this exercise.

• Begin by settling into a comfortable posture. Start to disengage the mind from busy thoughts and ideas. Close your eyes softly. Gently gather all your attention into the centre of your body. Try to reel in all thoughts that take you to the outside world.

• Allow the outside world to gradually melt away and dissolve into empty space. Begin by bringing your attention to the area around the crown of your head and gradually work down through your body to the tips of your toes.

• Focus on the area around the crown of your head. Gradually focusing on this area, imagine that all the tension in the muscles gradually dissolves away. Then focus on the temples and forehead, imagining any tension headache or pain dissolving away, disappearing as you place your mind on this part of the body – imagine the tension draining down through your body into the ground.

- All the tension in your head drains down through your body into the ground. Then imagine the tension in your jaw and ears gradually melting away – as you place your mind on this area, imagine any tension draining down through your body into the ground. Pause for a short while and then think to yourself my head is now comfortable and relaxed. Gently work your way down the body, relaxing each part and letting the tension drain away.

- Focus on the area of tension around your neck and shoulders. Try to relax the shoulders... lift them up gently and as they drop, imagine all the tension dissolving down into the ground; do this several times. As you do this, try to feel that any tension or weight that you are carrying in your shoulders melts away... feel as though you are really letting go of all the tension that is being held in your shoulders.

- Think to yourself, *my neck and shoulders are now comfortable and relaxed*. Relax your arms and hands, imagining all the tension in these areas draining out of your fingertips and far into the distance. Focus on the back and bring your mind to the top of the spine; focus on any area of tension that may have built up around the spine. Place your mind on these areas of tension and allow the knots to unravel as you focus on them and the tension dissolves down your spine out through the soles of your feet, into the ground.

- Mentally work your way down the spine, slowly relaxing and unravelling all the knots of tension and stress that may have built up. As your attention reaches the base of the spine, think to yourself now my back is comfortable and relaxed. Bring your attention to the front of your body; focus on the chest area and stomach. Try to identify any areas of stress or tension in this part of your body. Imagine that all the tension drains away, disappearing as you focus on it – imagine that any fear, tension or stress that have built up within the stomach disappear...

- Then think to yourself, now my chest and stomach are comfortable and relaxed. Then focus on your legs and feet, imagining any tension in these areas draining away, disappearing out of the soles of the feet – leaving you feeling comfortable and relaxed. Gradually scan down from the crown of your head to the tips of your feet, checking to see if there is any tension left in your body. If you locate any, then engage in the simple exercise presented above, again on that particular part of the body.

- Imagine all the tension drains out of your body and enjoy this experience of relaxation for a short time. You can think to yourself, my entire body is comfortable and relaxed. Gradually bring your relaxation to a close, by becoming aware of your body, and your position in the room. Gently open your eyes.

Key mindfulness ideas to consider using with young people

Special breathing

Deep breathing is nature's way of relaxing the brain and the body. You can distract the brain with controlled deep breathing. Get your children to inhale for the count of five. Hold the breath for a second, and then slowly exhale for a count of eight. Repeat ten times, or until calm.

Mindful doodling

Explain to the children that this doodling is special and will help them to remember what they've been taught during the day. It relaxes the mind, and allows the learning to make connections in the brain. It will also help if you play relaxing meditation music in the background.

Mindful gratitude

Throughout the day, get the children to stop, take three mindful breaths, and silently write down one thing they are thankful for, on a special gratitude list. By the end of the day, the list will be long and filled with happy thoughts. Send it home with the pupils to share with their families.

Worry stones

This is a 'focus object' that can allow children to release their worries and connect with their inner mindfulness of calm and peace. Have a collection of smooth stones to hand. When the child starts to become anxious, have them rub the stone, while focusing on the feel of the stone, and taking deep breaths.

✍ Activity 4.4 Case illustration

A referral has been made to your team by a teacher at a primary school concerning Jake, an 8 year-old boy. His behaviour is described as out of control, with a refusal to comply with instructions and aggression towards other pupils. He comes from a well-off family who live in owner-occupied property where both parents work full time. An older sibling, Francesca, took a non-fatal overdose of paracetamol 11 months ago when she was 14 years old and was seen briefly by the nearest child and adolescent mental health service.

A report by the consultant psychiatrist said that Francesca had been seriously depressed for some time before the overdose. She has been prescribed antidepressant medication. The psychiatrist described the parents as rigid disciplinarians with a low level of warmth towards their children. The mother is believed to be an alcoholic and the father works 14-hour days regularly in his own business.

✎ Make a provisional plan of action involving interprofessional and multi-disciplinary working.

💬 Commentary

Interprofessional and multi-disciplinary working will be crucial to the success of this case. Already there are potentially three or four different agencies with the possibility of six different professionals involved: teacher and educational psychologist in school; psychiatrist and therapist from CAMHS; social workers from the children and family team; and community psychiatric nurses from the adult community mental health team.

Clarifying case management and staff lines of accountability early on could save embarrassment or more serious problems later on. Make sure who does what and when with whom is recorded in accordance with an agreed plan. The social worker in the children and family team is likely to be expected to be the key worker and co-ordinator.

Agreeing a provisional plan and noting the variety of hypotheses, interpretations or explanations for the behaviour of the children needs to be done skilfully with balance and respect for the diversity of opinion likely to be expressed. For example, a provisional diagnosis of ADHD in Jake needs to be thoroughly assessed because of the impact such a label might have on all the stakeholders involved. The hard part is to match these ideas with what is required in terms of support or therapy, and whether the resources are there to provide it. Issues of gender and culture need to be openly addressed in terms of the family process and the tasks for different professionals.

The parents are crucial allies in this work. They must be engaged and encouraged to actively participate in planning and any work such as individual work with the children, family therapy, parent education or marital counselling. They may have fixed ideas about what is needed and shy away from marital counselling, so that may need to be kept as part of a later intervention as the case's natural history unfolds. They have seen medication work with Francesca and may press for the same medication to be prescribed for Jake.

Quick results are achievable, particularly if there is a lot of activity from a variety of professionals. However, the temptation may be to close the case and move on to other urgent work; however, this may disguise the fact that underlying problems may have simply been covered up in the light of attention paid to the children and the reduction in the level of anxiety. Keeping professionals and families engaged at these points is difficult, but an argument for prevention of further difficulties could succeed. Sometimes though, it is useful to have laid the foundation for families to alter their perception of themselves. This could avert a future crisis by enabling them to recognise the warning signs and seek help earlier.

Summary of key points

- The same intervention could be given to two children with the same problem, but only one of them might benefit. These dilemmas are important to acknowledge and reflect upon before proceeding with any course of action. The crucial point is to ensure the *most* effective intervention is offered for the *appropriate* problem with the *right* child.

- Practitioners working in an empowering or participatory way will strive to find, or offer themselves as, the most acceptable and accessible type of intervention resource. However, dilemmas will present themselves when some parents and/or children and young people express rigid views about what they want against the best available evidence of what can help.

- Some planning decisions will require breaking down into their component parts and being given careful consideration. But because this involves issues of uncertainty and values, intuition needs to be used within analysis in the making of judgements about the significance of information. Combining the explicitness of analysis with the skilled judgements of professional intuition offers you the advantages of each approach.

- Studies examining the efficacy of interventions tend to occur in clinical settings under controlled conditions. They do not therefore match with the practice reality for staff in non-specialist contexts undertaking several different roles. However, they serve a very useful purpose in providing knowledge and information about how mental health problems can be tackled. Many interventions and the theoretical base informing them are the same across a number of professional groups.

Further reading

Burton, M, Pavord, E and Williams, B (2014) ***An Introduction to Child and Adolescent Mental Health***. London: Sage.

Fonagy, P, Cottrell, D, Phillips, J, Bevington, D, Glaser, D and Allison, E (2016) ***What Works for Whom? Second Edition: A Critical Review of Treatments for Children and Adolescents***. New York: Guilford Press.

Joy, I, van Poortvliet, M and Yeowart, C (2008) *Heads Up: Mental Health of Children & Young People*. London: New Philanthropy Capital.

Luke, N, Sinclair, I, Woolgar, M and Sebba, J (2014) *What Works in Preventing and Treating Poor Mental Health in Looked After Children?* London: NSPCC.

McDougal, T (2016) *Children and Young People's Mental Health: Essentials for Nurses and Other Professionals*. London: Routledge.

McLaughlin, C and Holliday, C (2013) *Therapy with Children and Young People*. London: Sage.

Internet resources

Understanding Childhood: **www.understandingchildhood.net**

Meditation: **www.meditationinschools.org**

Mental Health Foundation: **www.mentalhealth.org.uk**

Chapter 5: How to help teenagers and parents understand each other

Introduction

Some young people feel that professional help is not for them, either because they may have experienced this at other times in their lives or they have seen professionals involved with parents or other family members and had a negative experience. Or it may be that they have heard stories from friends, or been raised in families where it is shameful, embarrassing or bad news to have professionals involved in your life. Some parents resent interference in what they believe to be their right to bring children up their way, or they mistrust the intentions of professionals, or they themselves may have had bad experiences when they were young people in which professionals did more harm than good.

Enabling young people and parents to communicate and manage the mental health problem is one of the best ways of helping and supporting the young person. Sometimes parents can feel undermined by professional involvement in their child's life, or they may be at their wit's end and desperate for outside help. It is a fine judgement to gauge the level, length and depth of your intervention. It is essential to maintain communication with everyone while respecting the young person's right to confidentiality. Some parents will feel offended that you don't tell them everything their child is saying to you if you are offering one-to-one support, while others will be happy and trust your professionalism and ethics.

At some point a young person may disclose sexual abuse happening to them within the family. They are more likely to feel safe doing this knowing they have a confidential relationship with you and that your primary job is to protect their interests above all others. Safeguarding procedures and protocols have developed in recent years so you should be able to access information and advice from your safeguarding manager about how to proceed in such circumstances. If you are a parent faced with the knowledge that another family member is abusing your child, you may be plunged into a state of shock, disbelief, denial, anger and guilt and may despair to the point you lash out at the child or even suggest they are lying. Young people very rarely lie about this; they are more likely to hide the truth under threats from the abuser or fear of the consequences of telling. Adult survivors nowadays are able to come forward and tell their stories thanks to wider understanding, awareness and the bravery of young people disclosing extremely traumatic experiences.

In other circumstances, your work as a professional may involve spending some time with parents/carers to help them understand the effects that stress and modern life is having on this generation of young people. A very useful technique is to enable them to reflect on their own teenage years – get them to chat to each other about what it was like growing up, ask them what stressed them, how did their parents help, who was helpful outside the family? This can be powerful and evoke quite an emotional response but it can help the process of them understanding their own child, recognising similarities and differences and fostering a sense of empathy.

What is stress?

Stress has become the widely used term among young people when they are seeking a word to express how they are feeling about something that is troubling or worrying them. In its early stages, stress is a response at a physical level which involves the body producing the chemicals adrenalin and cortisol, which make the heart beat faster, breathing rate increase and blood surge to the muscles. This prepares the body to fight or flee from a threat. Modern threats do not usually require this physical state, but anxiety or panic attacks about exams or relationships, abuse, parents fighting, bullying or long-term physical illness can produce a build-up in those chemicals which can harm the immune system. Some stress and anxiety is not a problem but prolonged or constant episodes need to be reduced.

What are the symptoms of stress?

- Difficulty sleeping.

- A feeling of tightness in the chest.

- Negative thoughts that won't go away.

- Persistent headaches.

- Loss of appetite.

- Mood swings.

- Biting fingernails.

- Not being able to concentrate.

- Feeling anxious and panicky.

What is troubling young people today?

There are specific factors that affect young people that it is important parents/carers are aware of. As they get older, children learn about the wider world around them and news reporting tends to focus on war, disaster, human suffering, murders and rapes, and environmental changes. These are frightening things. Young people are faced with greater demands not just from exams and pressures to perform highly, but also in terms of being expected to look ahead and plan their futures in work or college. It's also a time when deaths, bereavements and sad things affecting family or friends happen more so than in childhood. This can affect some young people deeply. Social media is notoriously difficult and young people feel pressure to engage with it but can find it disturbing and harmful. This is part of feeling forced to impress friends, gain their approval and conform to images of perfection (often fake and unattainable). Finally, hormone changes increase rapidly during this phase of their lives, causing physical changes which may feel too fast or too slow and mood swings resulting in angry outbursts, tearfulness and depression. Preparing parents for these issues or explaining them while they are emerging can enable understanding and empathy.

Relationship issues

Helping parents or carers appreciate that the teenage years are a time of rapid changes while at the same time relationships with friends can intensify, end or become complicated is useful in enabling mutual understanding. Moving to secondary school is stressful because it can mean losing old friends and making new ones, placing an emphasis on social skills that may be undeveloped, causing frustration and anxiety. This is a notoriously challenging time which can trigger mental health problems to erupt. Young people will begin to form opinions about their community, lifestyles, politics, social attitudes and each other. Or they may have some mutual friends who fall out with each other, raising issues of loyalty and pressure to pick sides in disputes. It is a time of the start of sexual attraction, which some young people feel stronger than others. A peer group may discuss this issue and create a pressure to engage in sexual activity, or an intimate friend may want to have sex against the wishes of the other. Attitudes and knowledge is available extensively, there are legal boundaries as to when sex is permitted, and there is a huge variety of familial, cultural and religious differences in what is acceptable or permissible sexual activity for young people.

Shyness and feelings of inadequacy can easily occur at this time, especially for young people who don't fit the misleading and unrepresentative body images found in the media. Many boys watch online pornography which usually features girls in submissive, masochistic roles, and as a result may develop unrealistic expectations of what a girlfriend will do. Young people need help and guidance to support them through these challenging times, with a trusted person who can listen, not judge, empathise and be available when a crisis might blow up. If a young woman becomes pregnant and does not want to continue the pregnancy, they will feel considerable stress and anxiety. They may feel ashamed and hide their situation, ignore it and go into denial, or fear the reaction of their parents/carers. Specific advice is available from specialist health professionals, school nurses and youth services in the statutory and voluntary sectors. If a young person doesn't want sex but someone forces them physically or by threats, or without consent, then it is rape. It is also rape if a young person was drunk or using drugs that prevented them giving consent. Here are some simple ideas to get across.

- Stay true to yourself, what you believe and want.

- Stick with people you respect.

- Do what genuinely feels right for you.

- Don't give in to pressure from people you don't respect.

- Value your self-esteem.

Alcohol and drugs: a cause or symptom of mental health problems?

Alcohol and drugs have never been more widely available or as cheap as they are now. Young people can be influenced by advertising, parent behaviour or peer pressure to experiment with alcohol and drugs. They may also be used to self-medicate to deal with feelings of anxiety and depression. Regular use of alcohol and drugs may also cause mental health problems to be triggered. It is part of the emerging independence and desire to be adult that fosters risk-taking and rebelliousness. For a short time, using drugs and alcohol can make some young people feel confident, happy and relaxed. But the consequences can include having an accident or causing an accident, becoming ill or addicted, or possibly death from an overdose or allergic reaction.

✎ Activity 5.1

Consider ways in which you dealt with stress when you were a teenager. Who was most helpful and what things worked for you?

⬭ Commentary

Depending on the type of stress and its frequency, the idea of taking a break or encouraging a young person to give themselves a reward is a good starting point. It means they have choices and are empowered to take charge of a situation which might feel hopeless. Things like drinking water frequently is known to be good for the body, as is having a healthy snack. Listening to music, lighting a scented candle or developing breathing exercises or meditation techniques is known to lower the heart rate. Being outdoors can help hugely, walking around looking at nature or engaging in sport is beneficial. Some young people find relaxation in reading or creative writing, cooking, keeping a scrapbook or photo album. A simple first aid breathing exercise involves the young person finding a quiet place to sit or lie down. Then they take six breaths in and then eight breaths out. While doing this, encourage them to move from the feet to the head concentrating on relaxing every major muscle, limb, neck, shoulders, jaw, fingers and toes.

When does anxiety resulting from stress become a problem?

Distressing: If relatively normal activities such as socialising or completing homework, or speaking to a class cause short-term anxiety, then this is different to a young person who becomes intensely anxious frequently, to the extent that it bothers them they get into such a state.

Duration: Most anxieties come and go, are short term and can be healthy to enable young people to cope with challenges. But if anxiety becomes ongoing and repetitive across a range of activities and situations then this makes it problematic.

Disproportionate: If a young person is facing an exam in a topic which they feel less confident in, then some anxiety will be generated. But if they feel anxious even with a topic they excel at and in other activities that other young people cope with, then this is a sign that their experience is disproportionate.

Disrupting: Normal anxiety can be protective but if it starts interfering with a young person's life in general, stops them socialising or attending school, or concentrating on simple tasks, then it may lead them to withdraw and feeling isolated from friends. Such disrupting anxiety is excessive and requires help and support to manage and overcome.

What is resilience?

Resilience is the capacity to 'bounce back' from adversity. Protective factors increase resilience, whereas risk factors increase vulnerability. Resilient individuals, families and communities are more able to deal with difficulties and adversities than those with less resilience. Those who are resilient do well despite adversity, although it does not imply that those who are resilient are unharmed – they often have poorer outcomes than those who have a low-risk background but less resilience. This applies to health outcomes and affects success in a range of areas of life across the life course. Evidence shows that resilience could contribute to healthy behaviours, higher qualifications and skills, better employment, better mental well-being, and a quicker or more successful recovery from illness.

Resilience is not an innate feature of some people's personalities. Resilience and adversity are distributed unequally across the population, and are related to broader socio-economic inequalities which have common causes – the inequities in power, money and resources that shape the conditions in which people live and their opportunities, experiences and relationships. Those who face the most adversity are least likely to have the resources necessary to build resilience. This 'double burden' means that inequalities in resilience are likely to contribute to health inequalities.

How to help build resilience in young people

Parents can help young people develop resilience because at its core it involves behaviours, thoughts and actions that can be learned over time. The following are ideas for building resilience.

• Help your child remember ways that they have successfully handled hardships in the past and then help them understand that these past challenges help them build the strength to handle future challenges. Help your child learn to trust himself or herself to solve problems and make appropriate decisions. Teach your child to see the humour in life, and the ability to laugh at oneself. At school, help children see how their individual accomplishments contribute to the well-being of the class as a whole.

• Even when your child is facing very painful events, help them look at the situation in a broader context and keep a long-term perspective. Although your child may be too young to consider a long-term outlook on their own, help them see that there is a future beyond the current situation and that the future can be good. An optimistic and positive outlook enables your child to see the good things in life and keep going even in the hardest times. In school, use history to show that life moves on after bad events.

• Tough times are often the times when children learn the most about themselves. Help your child take a look at how whatever they are facing can teach them that they have talent, skills and resources within them, which emerge when needed. At school, consider leading discussions of what each student has learned after facing down a tough situation.

- Change often can be scary for young people. Help your child see that change is part of life and that new goals can replace goals that have become unattainable. At school, point out how students have changed as they progress and discuss how that change has had an impact on them.

- Teach your child how to make friends, including the skill of empathy, or feeling another's pain. Encourage your child to be a friend in order to get friends. Build a strong family network to support your child through their inevitable disappointments and hurts. At school, watch to make sure that one child is not being isolated. Connecting with people provides social support and strengthens resilience. Some find comfort in connecting with a higher power, whether through organised religion or privately and you may wish to introduce your child to your own traditions of worship.

- Children who may feel helpless can be empowered by helping others. Engage your child in age-appropriate volunteer work, or ask for assistance yourself with some task that they can master. At school, brainstorm with children about ways they can help others. Maintaining a daily routine can be comforting to children, especially younger children who need structure in their lives. Encourage your child to develop their own routines.

- Explain how they can focus on something besides what's worrying them. Be aware of what your child is exposed to that can be troubling, whether it be news, the internet or overheard conversations, and make sure your child takes a break from those things if they trouble them. Although schools are being held accountable for performance on standardised tests, build in unstructured time during the school day to allow children to be creative.

- Help your child appreciate the importance of making time to eat properly, exercise and rest. Make sure your child has time to have fun, and make sure that your child hasn't scheduled every moment of their life with no 'down time' to relax. Caring for oneself and even having fun will help your child stay balanced and better able to deal with stressful times.

- Encourage your child to set reasonable goals and then to move towards them one step at a time. Moving towards that goal – even if it's a tiny step – and receiving praise for doing so will focus your child on what they have accomplished rather than on what hasn't been accomplished, and can help build the resilience to move forward in the face of challenges. At school, break down large assignments into small, achievable goals for younger children, and for older children, acknowledge accomplishments on the way to larger goals.

Family counselling/therapy as a way of enabling communication

Psychiatrists and psychologists discovered in the mid-twentieth century that instead of working with disturbed young people individually, they could gain better and quicker positive results by seeing the whole family together. They reported better outcomes when they worked with the whole family rather than the individual patient. The central theoretical idea informing this approach is that the symptomatic behaviour of a family individual is part of the transactional pattern peculiar to the family system in which it occurs. Therefore, the way to change the symptom is to change the rules of the family.

The goal of this way of working is to discover the current family rules and traditional ideas which sustain the potentially dysfunctional patterns of relating within the family. Change is achieved by clarifying the ambiguity in relationships that occur at a nodal point in the family's evolution such as a young person's emerging independence or exit from the home combined with the increase in responsibilities for an older relative or grandparent. Family therapists do not work to a normative blueprint of how an ideal family should function; rather, they can fit this method to suit all types of family. This approach furthermore emphasises the importance of the underlying beliefs held by family members about the problem which is affecting a young person's mood and behaviour. It avoids blaming other members of the family by working on the basis that the actions of various family members are the best they can do. These are some of the key features:

- **Positive connotation:** this technique involves reflecting back to the family a positive reason for all their actions. This is supported by providing a rationale for why they behave as they do, and maintains the therapist in a non-judgemental stance. It places the family members on an equal footing, thus avoiding scapegoating of any individual, particularly a young person.

- **Hypothesising:** this is a way of bringing together all the available information prior to the family session and collating it into a coherent whole which is fully circular and systemic. In other words, it attempts to explain why the family have a problem. This unproved supposition is tentative and is used as the basis for guiding the family session. The task for the worker is to confirm or disprove the hypothesis and create a new one if necessary.

- **Circular questioning:** this unique style of questioning is both elegant and simple. It requires the worker to ask questions of one member about the relationship between two other family members. The family will not be used to communicating in this way and are placed in a position of having to speak freely about ideas they would normally keep to themselves. Differences in perception and distinctions in behaviour can be explored and discussed according to the interviewer's curiosity and hypothesis. Surprising and important new information can be produced which every family member can hear and process.

• **Neutrality:** again, this is another distinguishing feature of family sessions. It involves the worker siding with everyone and showing no allegiance or favouritism to any individual family member. Although the worker may feel distinctly biased towards say, a victim of child abuse or domestic violence, the neutrality refers to behaviour during the interview rather than a moral injunction. The aim is to maximise the family's engagement and not collude in blaming behaviour which will undermine the desired change.

• **Intervention:** at the end of a family session, a prescription or intervention is delivered to all those present and can be mailed to any absent members. It can consist of a simple task or complex ritual designed to interrupt dysfunctional behavioural patterns and improve the mental health of the young person.

Brief family work

This approach is primarily aimed at a short-term period of work with the emphasis on solutions and encouraging families to recognise their own strengths and competencies. The mantra of practitioners using this way of working is 'focus on solutions not problems'. For example, a family or parents often discuss a child or a parent in sweeping generalisations when explaining their problems. 'He's always getting into trouble with teachers', or 'she never does as she is told'. These are recognisable complaints and express less the reality than an over-emphasis on the negative, as if the parents are trying to convince you of their case for help and their desperation. Solution-focused workers turn this idea around and carefully enable the complainants to recall an exception to this general rule about the troublesome child, person or event.

Once the family has recognised that exceptions do occur and the person can behave/do as they are asked, the focus of the approach is to emphasise these exceptions and help the family to make more of them happen. This requires patience and hard work to excavate every element surrounding these exceptions so that a family can prepare for them, recognise them, sustain them, and reproduce them. These are then translated into clear, recognisable goals that can be specifically described so that everyone involved can perceive them. Goal setting can often be difficult, especially with parents/families with poor self-esteem, lacking in confidence, and feeling disempowered. To help overcome this difficulty, the *miracle question* is designed to help families identify specific behaviours and actions that indicate change, rather than talk abstractly about wanting to 'be happy again', or 'be like a normal family'.

The miracle question entails asking the family to imagine that while they were all asleep a miracle happened and the problem was solved. When they awoke they were not aware a miracle had happened. They then have to describe what is different that tells them a miracle has occurred. In describing the difference, they are encouraged to make concrete the conditions for change and by doing so are in fact illustrating the goals they desire. The practitioner's job is to work collaboratively with the family's *own definition of change* and help them devise ways of achieving it. Overall, the brief solution-focused approach can be summarised in terms of three rules.

• **If it ain't broke don't fix it:** even the most chronic of problems show periods where the troublesome patterns or symptoms are absent or reduced. The worker needs to have a broad and tolerant view of what is not broke – what are the competencies? These can be built upon so that the work does not become bogged down into attempting to build the pursuit of an 'ideal' family.

• **Once you know what works, do more of it:** once exceptions and competencies have been discovered, then families are encouraged to do more of these. This can lead to a self-reinforcing cycle of success which will start to replace that of failure, incompetence and desperation.

• **If it doesn't work, don't do it again; do something different:** families often become involved in cycles where they cannot see any alternative but to continue to act in the ways they always have, or do more of the same. Searching for the exception, they can be helped to notice that an alternative pattern happens occasionally with more positive consequences. This is built upon until it replaces the previous more common negative pattern.

✎ Activity 5.2

🔦 Examine closely what are for you the core elements of this way of working, and then discuss these with a colleague.

🔦 Together, think about a young person you are trying to help and plan how you might try to arrange family sessions.

Changing families in modern society

Studies have detected intrafamilial changes in traditional patterns of kinship relationships and contact and support, where significant numbers of families have lost touch or were unable to rely on help when it was needed. Further complexity is revealed by research into subgroups of the population which, although sparse, offers evidence of the nature and variety of contemporary family life (Bhui and McKenzie, 2008). For example, while all ethnic groups had high levels of contact with non-resident parents, Asian and African-Caribbean people had higher levels of contact with aunts and uncles. The potential of other family members and grandparents to serve as helpful resources is indicative of a need for the widening of the focus in order to assess strengths within the wider family constellation and work preventively. Attention to culture and ethnicity as crucial influences on the interactional style and structure of families is important. Here are some key ideas to help in your work.

- Appreciate that within the majority culture there is no homogeneous group.

- Be aware of the subtleties of your own ethnic and cultural make-up and how this impacts upon your work.

- Avoid making assumptions about the internal structure of a family from their known culture, as defined by crude stereotypes or lazy generalisations.

Studies show that British Asian or American Asian families are like all other families, like some other families, and like no other families. It is suggested that cultural sensitivity can be learned and understood if culturally important values for this group are looked at. What follows here are, however, some generalisations for the sake of brevity, but we must always remember that each family is unique and requires an individual approach. The need for careful, reflective assessment and high-quality supervision before any intervention is made is vital.

As the volume and complexity of family problems increases, there is concern that the voluntary and non-governmental sectors will be unable to match the level of skills to the level of need expressed. Therefore, creative ways of thinking are generating effective resources, such as the family group conference approach to child welfare. Developed in New Zealand, it is based on a cultural-religious Indigenous concept among Maori people emphasising the relationship between celestial and terrestrial knowledge. According to Maori belief, the origin of the family group conference was a rebellious initiative by the children of *Ranginui*, the great Sky Father, and *Papatuanuku*, the matriarch Earth Mother.

Protected in a darkened cocoon by their parents, the children desired freedom to explore the outer limits of the universe. So the whole community or village was enlisted to help navigate this family problem. The family conference subsequently

Supporting Troubled Young People

convened included close and distant relatives and grandparents, all of whom were regarded as part of a single spiritual and economic unity. Thus, each Maori child's cultural identity is explicitly connected to their genealogy or *whakapapa*. The family group conference has been incorporated into mainstream services in the UK and elsewhere, where extended family members, especially grandparents, are invited to participate in care planning and become part of the family support system rather than excluded from it.

There is a long tradition in Asian culture of solving problems through mediation rather than using head-on confrontations. Family support staff are in a good position to mediate within a family's conflict because of their position of authority, knowledge of family relationships and use of techniques that can enhance face-saving with Asian families. In this situation, meeting with family members separately is suggested since airing their difficulties together at the outset may be too confrontational. This is in contrast to the suggestion of the importance of beginning family work with whole families.

This highlights how every family situation needs an individual appraisal by staff on receiving referrals to assess whether standard procedures, whatever those are in a particular agency, are appropriate for the particular family referred. The task of convening and engaging with that family will therefore vary, though it will remain the case that simply understanding the various parts of the family will not enable an understanding of the whole family and the individual contact will need to prepare family members for a family meeting.

American and British children who misbehave are often 'grounded'. Their punishment is to be forced to be with their family and it seems that one of the results of grounding is that children will fight their way out of the family (a process that Americans call emancipation). With Asian children, being excluded from the family is extremely rare and is viewed as a severe punishment. Thus, if children misbehave they are threatened with banishment from the family and told to get out. These children will have to fight to stay in the family and the expectation will be that they will remain within the family and will also bring their spouses to join it.

The point here is that neither approach is better or worse, simply that they are different and need to be understood before we try to intervene. An intervention based on the wrong premise for 'grounding' would otherwise totally fail and as workers we would be perplexed by this if we have assumed majority-culture norms. Indeed, with any family these expectations should be checked thoroughly.

The systems model of a careful, systematic assessment of how a family organises itself in relation to the necessary tasks of family life is particularly appropriate for understanding the uniqueness of any family. It enables workers to spend a number of sessions with each family, exploring their interaction patterns in a structured way before embarking on ideas and strategies aimed at encouraging change. It is also a model which focuses on our role as facilitators, working in partnership with a family and enabling or empowering family members rather than instructing or directing them.

What if a young person cannot talk to their parent(s)?

This is not uncommon in situations where a young person for whatever reason is not able to communicate with a parent and not willing to attend family sessions. This could be due to the adult's own mental illness, drug and alcohol abuse, a poor relationship, or the young person may want to protect them from becoming upset. If this is the case then a trusted adult needs to be available and a young person encouraged to talk with them. This could be a teacher, youth worker, social worker, the parent of a close friend, or a GP. A death in the family such as a grandparent can trigger strong feelings for every generation in a family. A young person faced with their own parent's grief and reaction to the death of their parent will simultaneously be feeling sad and mournful about the loss of a grandparent.

The death of a pet can be just as painful as the death of a human and should not be dismissed or downplayed in its significance. Both the parent and child may be so overwhelmed in their own grieving process that they find it hard to be emotionally available to each other. Due to their personality or level of maturity, the young person may feel it is their job to console their parent, while setting aside their own emotions. It could work the other way round if, for example, there was a particularly close bond between a grandparent and grandchild. Holding feelings in is not healthy in the long run and those feelings may get expressed in negative or destructive ways or behaviour. These are situations where an impartial, trusted outsider can engage with a young person and provide the comfort and support not available from the parent or carer. There are also online resources, some designed and run by young people themselves, which may be preferable to some young people rather than a face-to-face meeting. Here is a selection:

Childline: www.childline.org.uk

Runaway Helpline: www.runawayhelpline.org.uk

The Mix: www.themix.org.uk

Young Minds: https://youngminds.org.uk/find-help

How to engage young people using fables, legends and fairy stories

Children and young people have the capacity to conjure feelings of faith and hope when experiencing emotional and psychological distress. Myths, legends and fairy stories as part of their early child development offer a rich source of material to draw from and enlist in supporting young people. Fairies often act in a healing capacity in mythology, or they appear as agents between the world of human affairs and the invisible forces of nature. They also possess powers in advance of mortals achieving superhuman tasks, but they can also run into trouble and sometimes rely on assistance from humans to succeed. These tales contain metaphors and symbolic places or characters which can resonate with a young person facing confusion, internal conflict or frightening feelings.

A sample of tales from a variety of countries shows how we can discern some common themes as well as unique stories – it is a delicious cultural mixture and reflective of the reservoir of material available to us in our work for use with the children and young people we are hoping to heal in some way. Harnessing the child's imagination can be a powerful vehicle for a transforming experience at the psychic level. So what better way of accessing their imagination than by exploring memories of fairy stories and using them to address painful or unsettling issues in a non-threatening, playful manner?

These childhood stories are often experienced as bedtime reading or spoken by a parental/carer figure. They are usually extraordinary tales involving fantastical characters and situations where magic is woven in a world outside the physical daily world inhabited during the waking day. Good and evil usually feature in a struggle during trials and tribulations; morality also features and happy endings are the preferred outcome. Before printed books, these myths and legends were part of narrative communication; storytelling was a vital part of entertainment as well as education. Beneath this classic literary device perhaps lies a desire for a positive outcome, a hopeful belief or a basic trust in such a thing as natural justice. Many of our clients will have struggled so much precisely because these primitive notions have not stood the cruel test of reality. As victims of abuse or neglect they will have experienced the triumph of evil over good rather than the other way round. In addition to the repertoire of helping techniques available within a variety of counselling or therapeutic modes, enabling a young person to identify with a fairy tale or to make their own version up could be a useful means of unlocking feelings of mistrust or guilt.

Towards deeper cultural meaning

As part of the healing process, literature is an often underrated asset. Yet it carries information about families, emotions, morality, relationships and so much else in a way that can enable very damaged children to use devices such as fairy stories to help understand themselves at a deeper level. Fairy stories have the capacity to capture the child's imagination because they usually involve fantastical creatures, transformational experiences or complex predicaments in which the child can immerse themselves and relate to their inner world. It is there that a child's repressed feelings and worst fears lurk, causing inner conflicts that manifest in acting out behaviour or anxiety states. The fairy story operates at the overt level where obvious concepts of right and wrong and other moral dilemmas are struggled with. It also operates at a covert level carrying important messages to the conscious, preconscious and unconscious mind that affect the child's sense of culture.

By tackling head on the basic human predicaments of life, death and the meaning of existence, the fairy story is an economical means for children and young people to access these crucial issues and confront them in a symbolic form. They are a simplified story reduced to the bare essentials with few details and typical characterisations. For example, many fairy stories begin with the death of a parent figure – thereby capturing instantly the central fear and at times the fantasy wish of every child. Dualities of good and evil are equally the most common theme in fairy stories where the eternal struggle takes place through many trials and tribulations. With the usual triumph of good over evil, the child is thereby able to identify with the symbolic figure and absorb the moral message internally.

The important role of grandparents

With changing family patterns, increased life expectancy, growing numbers of dual-worker households and higher rates of family breakdown, grandparents are now playing an increasing role in their grandchildren's lives. They can be a critical yet overlooked resource in supporting children with mental health problems. Contemporary grandparents and grandchildren see each other moderately frequently. In the UK, the British Social Attitudes (BSA) survey found that 30 per cent of grandparents reported seeing grandchildren several times a week; conversely, 32 per cent said they saw their grandchild less than once a month (NatCen, 2017). The relationship is usually (though not invariably) quite close and satisfying, rather than conflictual, and is seen as positive and important by both generations. Just as mothers are more often the closer parent to children, many studies find that grandmothers are involved with their grandchildren more than grandfathers are. Also, grandparents through the mother's side are typically more involved than those through the father's side.

Grandparents and grandchildren do all sorts of things together, such as taking part in family events, having treats, imparting family history, playing games, going on holidays, shopping, watching TV or videos, babysitting, giving emergency help, giving personal advice, joining in religious activity, and giving advice on school. The BSA survey found that trips to the park or playground tended to make way for indoor games or watching TV at around the age of six. Research from Gohilipour (2013) reports conversations as being prominent in activities reported by Polish grandchildren. Because they are close but do not have a parental authority role, grandparents can act as confidants in situations where an older child might not wish to confide in a parent. Also, grandparents will often know more about family history.

How to challenge stereotypes

Television and children's books often portray grandparents as aged, fussy, domesticated and sedentary, probably with infirmities (Roald Dahl is a culprit in this respect), although this is beginning to change. The stereotype is out of step with demographic realities, as most grandchildren who read children's books will have grandparents in their forties to sixties. For most people, becoming a grandparent is a positive experience; but this can depend on the age at which it happens. Nearly one-third of grandparents enter grandparenthood 'off-time': either before 40 or after 60.

Research with black African/Caribbean grandmothers (Gohilipour, 2013) found that those women who became grandmothers early (35–37 years) were discontented, experiencing obligations they were not ready for. They were also affected by the negative stereotypes associated with grandparenting and age.

What influence can grandparents have on development?

Influences can be direct, resulting from contact and face-to-face interaction, and indirect, mediated by other means such as parental behaviour. One source of the indirect influence of grandparents is via financial support. Also, by acting as parents themselves, grandparents influence how their children act as parents. It has been found that there is 65 per cent concordance in attachment security across three generations: maternal grandmothers' and mothers' adult attachment status and infants at 12 months (Sette et al, 2015).

Attachment theory emphasises consistency over generations, but it also predicts that adults can work through or resolve unsatisfactory relations with their parents and modify their internal working models, either through self-reflection or with the aid of therapy or counselling. Many survivors of the Holocaust in the Second World War (now grandparents) score unresolved on the Atlantoaxial Instability (AAI), due to the traumatic way in which they lost their parents at an early age; but few of their children score unresolved, and their grandchildren appear to be indistinguishable from the remaining population in terms of attachment characteristics.

Research on children's anti-social behaviour from Rutter et al (2008) also points to intergenerational influences. The use of physically aggressive and punitive techniques in the grandparent/parent generation predicts similar behaviour in the parent/grandchild generation, and also anti-social behaviour in the grandchildren. Examples of direct influence are giving gifts, being a companion and confidant, acting as an emotional support or 'buffer' at times of family stress, passing on family history or national traditions, and acting as a role model for ageing. Workers with families of Bangladeshi origin in the East End of London found examples of synergistic learning interactions between grandparents and grandchildren; the grandmother would help the grandchild learn about their Bengali language and heritage, while the grandchild would be helping their grandmother learn how to use computers and speak English (Walker, 2016).

Childcare

Regular childcare from grandparents can provide help for the middle generation. The BSA survey found that about one-fifth of grandparents looked after grandchildren once a week or more; this was almost as common for children aged 5 to 12 (after-school or holiday care) as for pre-school children, and was more frequent when mothers were working part time, than full time. Grandchild care can later lead to close grandparent/grandchild relationships. Many grandparents enjoy looking after a grandchild, which can be an opportunity for indulging them. But some grandmothers, especially paternal grandmothers, may be reluctant to provide long-term support of childcare for working mothers.

In parent-maintained households with co-resident grandparents there is much greater opportunity for helping with childcare. Although this is more the norm in some traditional societies, in grandparent-maintained households, the grandparents are actually responsible for their grandchildren. In many such cases there are family problems and poverty, and research from Freer (2016) finds that grandchildren reared in grandparent-headed households have poorer academic performance than similar children in parent-headed households, and that grandparents in grandparent-headed households have a higher incidence of depression and risk for physical and emotional health problems. Grandparents can experience unexpected difficulties if they wish to adopt grandchildren who lack parental care. However, the most debated legal aspects relating to grandparents concern access to grandchildren when parents divorce.

After relationship breakdown

When parents separate and divorce, the relationship of grandparents to parents, particularly to a custodial parent (or one who has care and control of the grandchildren) becomes a crucial issue. If these are harmonious, grandparents can provide stability, support and nurturance to the grandchild(ren) and family, often providing financial assistance or childcare. They can negotiate relationship difficulties between the parent and grandchild and be a 'buffer' during times of family distress. Closeness to maternal (but not paternal) grandparents was significantly associated with grandchild adjustment when parents had separated, even when other family variables were controlled for (Sette et al, 2015).

In contrast, a difficult or disrupted grandparent–parent relationship can threaten proximity of grandparents to grandchildren, contact, involvement and fulfilment of a satisfying grandparental role. If as is usually the case the children reside with their mother, then paternal grandparents may have to 'tread carefully' in obtaining access to their grandchildren; and it can be denied. The consequences of unwanted loss of contact with grandchildren can be devastating. Grandparents who were members of support groups such as the Grandparents Association reported symptoms of bereavement and negative effects on their physical and emotional health after loss of contact with their grandchildren due to parental divorce, more so than with separation just arising from geographical distance.

An important issue for grandparents is what access and visitation rights they have with grandchildren. Sometimes legal contact orders are the only way of obtaining these. Under the Children Act 1989, any person (not just grandparents or relatives) may seek leave to apply for an order for contact with a child. But even if the grandparent has obtained a contact order there is little that holds the parent to abide by the court ruling. The issue of what further legal rights grandparents should have continues to be debated.

The three-generation family relationships which can follow divorce are complex. A grandchild could have various types of step-grandparent, resulting from a parent remarrying (the most usual), a grandparent remarrying, or from the parent of a step-parent remarrying. The BSA survey found that step-grandparents generally had less contact with grandchildren than did grandparents; but an interesting finding was that step-grandfathers generally had more contact (20 per cent seeing step-grandchildren several times a week) compared with step-grandmothers (11 per cent) (NatCen, 2017).

⚒ Summary of key points

✦ Enabling young people and parents to communicate and manage the mental health problem is one of the best ways of helping and supporting the young person. Sometimes parents can feel undermined by professional involvement in their child's life, or they may be at their wits' end and desperate for outside help. It is a fine judgement to gauge the level, length and depth of your intervention.

✦ Stress has become the widely used term among young people when they are seeking a word to express how they are feeling about something that is troubling or worrying them. In its early stages, stress is a response at a physical level which involves the body producing the chemicals adrenalin and cortisol which make the heart beat faster, breathing increase and blood surge to the muscles.

✦ Resilience is the capacity to 'bounce back' from adversity. Protective factors increase resilience, whereas risk factors increase vulnerability. Resilient individuals, families and communities are more able to deal with difficulties and adversities than those with less resilience. Those who are resilient do well despite adversity, although it does not imply that those who are resilient are unharmed – they often have poorer outcomes than those who have a low-risk background but less resilience.

✦ Children and young people have the capacity to conjure feelings of faith and hope when experiencing emotional and psychological distress. Myths, legends and fairy stories as part of their early child development offer a rich source of material to draw from and enlist in supporting them.

✦ With changing family patterns, increased life expectancy, growing numbers of dual-worker households and higher rates of family breakdown, grandparents are now playing an increasing role in their grandchildren's lives. They can be a critical yet overlooked resource in supporting children with mental health problems.

Further reading

Carr-Gregg, M and Shale, E (2013) *Adolescence: A Guide for Parents*. Sydney: HarperCollins.

Cotterill, J (2016) *A Library of Lemons*. London: Templar Publications.

Fitzpatrick, C and Sharry, J (2004) *Coping with Depression in Young People: A Guide for Parents*. London: Wiley.

Public Health England (2014) *Local Action on Health Inequalities: Building Children and Young People's Resilience in Schools*. London: Public Health England.

Tompkins, M and Martinez, K (2010) *My Anxious Mind: A Teen's Guide to Managing Anxiety and Panic*. Washington, DC: Magination Press.

Walker, S and Akister, J (2004) *Applying Family Therapy: A Guide for Caring Professionals in the Community*. Lyme Regis: Russell House Publishers.

Whitaker, T and Fiore, D (2015) *Dealing with Difficult Parents*. London: Routledge.

Internet resources

Childline: **www.childline.org.uk**

Parents' information: **www.minded.org.uk**

Young Minds: **www.youngminds.org.uk**

Chapter 6: What are the current issues challenging young people?

Introduction

The Institute of Fiscal Studies (2011) calculates that relative child poverty in the UK is projected to rise by six percentage points between 2010 and 2020, from 17.5 per cent to 23.5 per cent, or over 1 million children. This will reverse all the fall in relative child poverty seen between 2000–1 and 2010–11. Absolute child poverty over the same period is projected to increase by 9.6 percentage points. Changes to the benefits system introduced by the government account for almost all of the increase in absolute child poverty projected over the next few years. Relative child poverty would actually have fallen in the absence of the changes.

Statistics from Campbell et al (2016) show that England and Wales imprisons more 14 year olds than any other European country. In Britain, at least one child dies each week as a result of adult cruelty. It has been estimated that about 5,000 minors are involved in prostitution in Britain at any one time. In 2017 there were about 390,000 children in need in England.

One-quarter of all rape victims are children and 75 per cent of sexually abused children do not tell anyone at the time. Each year about 30,000 children are on child protection registers. Recorded offences of gross indecency with a child more than doubled from 1985 to 2010, and in 2017 there were 46,352 offences but convictions against perpetrators actually fell from 42 per cent to 19 per cent. Fewer than one in 50 sexual offences results in a conviction, and there is still a major shortfall in the supervision and treatment of sexual offenders thus reducing the opportunity to reduce re-offending rates.

Young people are growing up in an increasingly turbulent world politically, economically and socially. This context is important for understanding the modern challenges unique to this generation. Experiencing adolescence might be better understood as navigating less a discrete event and more a period during which earlier difficulties that may have been either hidden or manageable hitherto become exposed or re-exposed under external stress and family pressures. If adolescence is turbulent largely because of the identity crisis elicited by physical, neurobiological and hormonal changes, one can suppose that a robust pre-adolescent sense of self will provide some protection. The pre-teen years (8–12 years) are increasingly understood to be a crucial time for the crystallisation of identity which, from about the age of eight, encompasses gender, social acceptability and competence.

Children take their view of themselves, informed by their treatment within the family, and test this on the world outside (friends, peers and teachers). Their stronger bodies and more reflective and capable minds provide the chance to improve their range of skills and competence. But if they have no mother or father on whom to model themselves, if their self-image at the start of this period is negative or is undermined during this important stage, if they have few opportunities to develop interests and skills that fuel pride or to practise autonomy, or if they have poor relationship and attachment experiences, then their ability either to do well in school or to form good friendships can be compromised, with potentially devastating consequences. Even those who have no special problems face more intense academic, social and financial pressures that can shake self-belief.

What is the future role of schools?

Late in 2017 the UK government published a Green Paper laying out their plans for children and young people's mental health services. The proposals include introducing mental health support teams (linked to groups of schools and colleges), designated leads for mental health in all schools, new guidance for schools that will address the effect of trauma and a four-week waiting time target across CAMHS. There is little detail about these proposals, especially whether promised funding will materialise, how schools will cope with extra responsibilities, and where new staff will be recruited from when there are high vacancy levels in CAMHS services and schools are suffering problems recruiting and retaining enough teachers. Teachers' unions and children's charities have described these plans as too little too late. The plans are for trailblazer pilot programmes to be offered in a small number of locations, meaning only 25 per cent of young people will have access to support in the next five years.

Self-harm in young people

What is self-harm?

Deliberate self-harm has been defined as *'causing deliberate hurt to your own body, most commonly by cutting, but also by burning, abusing drugs, alcohol or other substances'* (Laye-Ginghu and Schonert-Reichl, 2005). Another description is to call the problem self-injury: *'a way of dealing with difficult feelings, by cutting, burning or bruising, taking an overdose of tablets, pulling hair or picking skin'* (Bird and Falkener, 2000). Young people at risk of developing this problem are usually 14 year-old and older adolescents who are depressed, have low self-esteem or have been sexually abused.

The definition of self-harm is also associated with *attempted suicide, parasuicide, suicidal gestures* and *manipulative attempts*. These terms are widely used by a variety of health and welfare professionals and can lead to confusion for parents and those trying to help the troubled young person. Most young people with this problem are not actually attempting suicide in that they do not start off with a plan to end their own life.

But it is important when trying to understand this problem to distinguish between young people who want to die; those who do not want to die; and those who are ambivalent as to whether they die or not, in order to design the most effective way to help. Self-harm may help someone to cope with feelings that threaten to overwhelm them: painful emotions, such as rage, sadness, emptiness, grief, self-hatred, fear, loneliness and guilt. These can be released through the body, where they can be seen and dealt with.

Self-harm may serve a number of purposes at the same time. It may be a way of getting the pain out, of being distracted from it, of communicating feelings to somebody else, and of finding comfort. It can also be a means of self-punishment or an attempt to gain some control over life. Because they may feel ashamed, afraid, or worried about other people's reactions, people who self-harm often conceal what they are doing rather than draw attention to it.

How common is this problem?

Research in this area has only been conducted in recent years (Walker, 2012a) as the problem has come to the attention of more and more parents, teachers, social workers and all staff who are in regular contact with children and young people. According to figures from the Nuffield Trust (2018), in England and Wales in 2018 there were about 15,000 admissions to accident and emergency hospital departments as a result of deliberate self-harm. Since many acts of self-harm do not come to the attention of health care services, hospital attendance rates do not reflect the true scale of the problem. A recent national interview survey suggested that in Great Britain between 4.6 and 6.6 per cent (or 25,000) of young people have self-harmed. However, even this might be an underestimate. In a school survey, 13 per cent of young people aged 15 or 16 reported having self-harmed at some time in their lives and 7 per cent as having done so in 2017.

Many parents who are shocked and frightened will try to help their child themselves, try to access CAMHS or seek private help from counsellors/therapists. How each family reacts to and deals with the problem will have some bearing on how quickly the young person recovers and comes to terms with their actions. This means that matters can worsen, stay the same, or resolve quite quickly. For example, interrogating the young person or criticising them will only further lower their self-esteem; discussing how they feel and what can be changed to help them stop is better. As a professional you need to be sensitive to how parents/carers express their distress, so your communication needs to be carefully worded to avoid leaving the young person with burdensome guilt feelings.

Much will depend on the resilience and coping culture within the family. For example, how have previous individual problems been managed? Have they been hidden and 'swept under the carpet'? Are emotions easily expressed or bottled up prior to exploding? Is the family 'enmeshed' – so close and tight that there is too little time and space for individuals to exercise some free expression? Or is the family so fluid that they act as separate individuals, hardly communicating, eating separately, watching TV on their own?

There is no correct way for families to operate, but it is important that they, together with professional help, can understand how they function, communicate and interact in order to establish a baseline of where they are at. Awareness of this (which might come as a surprise to some family members) provides the context for change if that is desirable or even possible. Crucial to any success is to cancel any blaming, finger-pointing, or digging up old conflicts and accusations – this will only make matters worse and make it harder to gain success.

How to begin to assess self-harming behaviour

Some young people may self-harm just once or twice. For others it can become a habitual response to any overwhelming situation. They might self-harm several times per day during difficult periods in their life. Therefore, it is important that the issue is addressed immediately; assessment is the gateway to understanding and future management. It is rare for self-harming behaviour to exist in isolation. Self-harm often follows on from earlier problem behaviours and illustrates that an addictive quality may exist across a range of behaviour. The literature supports the view that for young women there are well-established links both with eating disorders and overdosing. Any risk assessment should be able to answer the following:

• What makes the person harm themselves?

• Do they want to die when they commit the act of self-harm?

• Have they felt this way before?

• Have they had any previous help with self-injurious behaviour?

- Do they still feel like harming themselves?

- Do they want help?

A risk assessment needs to be directed at four main issues: assessment and management of the current episode; identification and management of associated problems; identification and promotion of the child and family's resources; and prevention of repetition. It is important that plans developed from any assessment set clear goals, the first of which should be to avoid accidental death. The worker or parent/carer might usefully generate suggestions on what decisions might help end the self-harming behaviour.

One example might be to ensure that the young person spends a lot of time in public places so they do not isolate themselves. This might counter the risk of self-harm in privacy since this is usually the location for such an act. Other tasks might include having the young person examine the short-term advantages of self-harm with the long-term consequences (such as scars or accidental death).

Another important goal is to try to reduce environmental stress by slowly but surely increasing the young person's connection to parents, friends and peer groups to improve communication skills, develop effective measures of self-soothing that do not include self-harm, and improve mood and emotional regulation. As such, the identification of stressors within the home and school is an important part of the work, as is the plan to decrease such stressors. There are many useful ways to engage the young person in finding alternative coping mechanisms.

✑ Activity 6.1

What can parents do to encourage and reinforce different coping mechanisms?

💬 Commentary

Parents or carers can try to recommend that a young person avoids spending long periods on their own. Isolation can be perfectly reasonable as a way of shutting out harmful things but invariably young people rely on the internet and social media as a primary communication tool so they will encounter the bullying in that medium. Doing something creative such as painting can be a distraction plus an activity that requires a degree of concentration away from the bullying behaviour. Expressing emotions through art is a well-tried means of releasing painful feelings. There are many examples available for engaging in calming activities or relaxation exercises such as mindfulness, meditation, breathing techniques, yoga or listening to some soothing music. It's important that a young person is able to make time for activities that they enjoy, which they may have neglected or forgotten about while preoccupied and distracted by cyberbullies. Never underestimate the power of talking, and although they may feel reluctant it is important to encourage them to phone a supportive friend for a chat.

Sustaining support

It may take the young person a long time before they are ready to give up self-harm completely. They may even find that their need for it increases as they explore distressing experiences in their past that may underlie their self-harm or make changes in the way that they live their life. Try not to let them get discouraged. The more progress they can make in sorting out other areas of their life, the easier giving up self-harm will eventually become.

Although many parents/carers consider it irrational, it is important that professionals do not aggressively discourage the young person from engaging in acts of self-harm. Rules place restrictions on their freedom. When we maintain the right to choose, our choices are much more powerful and effective. Telling a young person to not injure her/himself is both aversive and condescending. Because self-harm is used as a method of coping and is often used as an attempt to relieve emotional distress when other methods have failed, it is essential for the person to have this option. Most young people would choose to not hurt themselves if they could.

Although self-harm produces feelings of shame, secrecy, guilt and isolation, it continues to be utilised as a method of coping. That young people will engage in self-harming behaviours despite the many negative effects is a clear indication of the necessity of this action to their survival. It is really important that support, and not limits, is offered to that young person. Self-harm should be viewed as a way of coping. While self-harm appears dangerous and destructive, it actually may be an attempt at self-healing or self-preservation. Many young people who self-harm are victims and are finding a coping mechanism for themselves.

As mentioned earlier, the role of parents and other close relatives is important in determining the progress of the young person to recovery. The crucial task for the professional involved is to closely support the parents/carers; this will empower them and restore their confidence in coping with and managing a very stressful situation. In turn, this will have a positive impact on the troubled young person. Clear and unconditional positive support will help the troubled young person enormously and the task of the professional is to help the adults understand that their help and support for their child can be simple and uncomplicated. This support may be very simple; for example, spending time with them and listening may seem to the parent/carer like they are not doing anything. In fact, being present, available and calm will help the young person much more than being intrusive, questioning and directive.

The internet and cyberbullying

Being bullied can have just as damaging an effect on a child as more apparently serious types of abuse. It can involve name-calling, threats, insults, hitting, kicking, cyberbullying and other violence – meaning it can be physically, emotionally and even sexually abusive. The most frequent bullying takes the form of name-calling and physical assault. Other ways in which children are bullied include gestures, extortion and exclusion from a friendship or peer group.

Adults such as parents, other family members and teachers also bully children. They may do it by making a child feel bad/embarrassed or humiliated in front of other people, by shouting, teasing or poking fun at them. Recent research by Walker (2012a) revealed that websites encouraging suicide and self-harm topped a list of teenagers' greatest worries about the internet. The findings have raised fears that growing numbers of young people are becoming vulnerable to the messages being put out by such sites. The findings came just a week after widespread condemnation of internet trolling associated with the death of the cyberbullying victim Amanda Todd. The Canadian teenager was found dead after she had posted a harrowing YouTube video in which she told of the online bullying she had suffered by holding up handwritten notes.

What is cyberbullying?

• The use of information and communication technologies such as email, mobile phone and pager text messages, instant messaging or defamatory personal websites.

• Repetitive, wilful or persistent behaviour intended to cause harm, carried out by an individual or a group; inappropriate text messaging and emailing; sending offensive or degrading images by phone or via the internet; gossiping; excluding people from groups and spreading hurtful and untruthful rumours.

• Blogs, online games and defamatory online personal polling websites, to support deliberate, repeated and hostile behaviour by an individual or group, which is intended to harm others.

Supporting Troubled Young People

Many school students involved in cyberbullying can be unaware of what they are contributing to. They may feel it is harmless fun, teasing or banter and be unaware that recipients can feel extremely upset by name-calling or embarrassing things being posted about them. School anti-bullying policies are not effective in stopping it because of the special nature of this form of bullying, which allows those involved in passing on hurtful material to feel less responsible. Very little research has been done to investigate the issue of cyberbullying, but more is emerging as the harmful impacts are being registered. It seems quite clear that it is as harmful if not more harmful than the usual forms of bullying due to the secret nature of the attack, and the invasion of personal space. Potentially harmful messages can be displayed to a large audience in minutes on a variety of social media platforms.

How prevalent is cyberbullying?

According to Walker (2012b), nearly one-third of all 11 to 16 year olds have been bullied online, and for 25 per cent of those the bullying was ongoing. Several recent studies confirm a worrying picture in which 18 per cent of students in Years 6 to 8 said they had been cyberbullied at least once in the last couple of months. Six per cent said it had happened to them two or more times.

Eleven per cent of students in Years 6 to 8 said they had cyberbullied another person at least once in the last couple of months and 2 per cent said they had done it two or more times. Nineteen per cent of regular internet users between the ages of 10 and 17 reported being involved in online aggression; 15 per cent had been aggressors, and 7 per cent had been targets; 3 per cent were both aggressors and targets. Seventeen per cent of 6 to 11 year olds and 36 per cent of 12 to 17 year olds reported that someone said threatening or embarrassing things about them in emails, instant messages, websites, chat rooms or text messages.

Cyberbullying has increased dramatically in recent years as technology, cameras and video smartphones increase their applications. In nationally representative surveys of 10 to 17 year olds, twice as many children and youth indicated they had been victims and perpetrators of online harassment in the past 10 years.

What is the impact of cyberbullying on mental health?

Research from Walker (2011b) enables us to be quite confident about the specific problems that result from cyberbullying as a consequence of the way an individual reacts to the chronic stress of being consistently involved in predictable, aggressive and humiliating situations. Reactions include not sleeping well, bed wetting, feeling sad,

Chapter 6: What are the current issues challenging young people?

121

experiencing headaches and having tummy aches. It has been estimated that between 15 and 25 young victims of cyberbullying commit suicide each year in the UK.

A precise number is difficult to quantify due to the way suicides among young people are officially recorded. Coroners are reluctant to record suicide without corroborating proof of intent such as a suicide note and out of genuine sensitivity to grieving relatives. The relationship between bullying or being bullied and low self-esteem is a striking feature of research studies (Walker, 2011b) in this particular aspect of bullying. It is more often assumed that the relationship between being bullied and low self-esteem is one of cause and effect. Most studies have been correlational in nature, meaning that the two tend to coincide. Thus, low self-esteem itself may elicit bullying from other children and that low self-esteem is both a cause and effect of cyberbullying.

Who does this and why?

The capacity to exit a location immediately after insulting or harming another may encourage these behaviours in otherwise placid individuals. Trolling on newsgroups or chat rooms in which a person deliberately makes inflammatory comments in order to provoke heated arguments is an example of an internet-specific anti-social behaviour. Flaming occurs when a person viciously berates someone in a social networking chat room, and is another familiar online activity associated with bullying. When these activities attract negative comments and disapproval, the perpetrator can avoid rebuke by logging off or deleting the critical comment on their social media device.

What are the implications?

As cyberbullying is more secretive than traditional bullying, perpetrators are not always aware of the immediate effects their behaviour has on the victim. As a result, cyberbullies might experience less empathy than those who bully in the traditional sense, indicating a need to strengthen assessment tools for early detection of potential cyberbullies.

✎ Activity 6.2

🖊 Consider what can be done in your work or home context to decrease cyberbullying.
🖊 Discuss and share your ideas with a friend or colleague and think about how to instigate change.

Supporting Troubled Young People

Commentary

The development of educational programmes initiated around improving awareness of cyberbullying for young people, parents/carers and schools needs to be stepped up. It is necessary to deliver education that brings together young people and their families to enhance communication in relation to online media, to understand its potential for good and bad behaviour and educate young people about what constitutes acceptable behaviour online. Measures and resources need to be developed in a public health context to support young people to report incidents of cyberbullying in confidence. Other young people could help change attitudes and provide a source of peer support to young people who are affected by cyberbullying. Social networking sites are complicit in the harm caused and require legal sanctions to be imposed upon them and punitive fines to force them to remove malicious content and supervise harmful behaviour much more rigorously. In CAMHS and other support services, therapeutic methods and models may require changing, adapting or enhancing to reflect the particular characteristics of both bullies and victims of cyberbullying and their needs. Or new methods and techniques may emerge that are more effective in deterring and treating those young people affected. Criminal prosecution is available using existing laws if an offender persists and is unresponsive to re-education and other efforts to change their behaviour. Public health and education policies and practice that take a holistic approach and which stress the importance of developing values of togetherness need to be designed, so that young people learn about compassion, empathy and co-operation and can be deterred from the selfish, materialistic, acquisitive culture they are immersed in. A wider culture of care and kindness among young people, rather than an ethos of competition and individuality, needs to be developed and implemented. This increasing problem requires urgent and sustainable action at the personal, family, community and government level, sooner rather than later. The digital world is contributing to the further isolation and self-centred context of the emotional and psychological development of young people. The long-term personal and social consequences are poor unless this problem is tackled meaningfully.

Attention deficit hyperactive disorder (ADHD)

ADHD is a neurodevelopmental disorder which is defined by behaviour. The major symptoms are impulsivity, hyperactivity and inattention. In the past decade, the number of young people diagnosed has increased dramatically, leading to debates about over-diagnosis and medication being used to manage normal boisterous behaviour. Children with the most common form are easily distracted and have difficulty controlling their attention, though they don't show hyperactive or compulsive behaviour. Those with the hyperactive-compulsive subtype show inappropriately high levels of physical activity and have difficulty controlling their behaviour in a way that is appropriate for their age. In order to get a diagnosis, symptoms must cause problems for the child and those around them in at least two settings, for example at home and at school.

Symptoms must also be present for at least six months between the ages of 6 and 12 years. So this disorder is intrinsically linked to the environment: it's about how behaviour is appropriate for a situation, as well as the impact that a child's behaviour has on a situation. ADHD management recommendations vary by country and usually involve some combination of counselling, lifestyle changes and medication. The British guideline only recommends medication as a first-line treatment in children who have severe symptoms and for it to be considered in those with moderate symptoms who either refuse or fail to improve with counselling. The British Psychological Society says that physicians and psychiatrists should not follow the American example of applying medical labels to such a wide variety of attention-related disorders (Frances, 2011). The idea that children who don't attend or who don't sit still in school have a mental disorder is not entertained by most British clinicians.

What is problematic about using teacher–parent perceptions to diagnose ADHD?

The British Psychological Society's response to DSM V, the latest diagnostic guidelines, had more concerns than plaudits about the value judgements that were being included in assessment criteria (Frances, 2011). It criticised proposed diagnoses as clearly based largely on social norms, with symptoms that all rely on subjective judgements by parents and teachers that are not value-free, but rather reflecting current normative social expectations. They also expressed a major concern that clients and the general public are negatively affected by the continued and continuous medicalisation of their natural and normal responses to their experiences. These demand helping responses, but do not reflect illnesses so much as normal individual variation. Publishing in *The Cochrane Library*, a group of scientists have reviewed the evidence around the effects of a common drug which is used to treat ADHD in children and adolescents, reporting that Methylphenidate (Ritalin) is associated with some benefits but also an increased risk of non-serious adverse effects (Punja et al, 2016).

Both children with and without ADHD abuse stimulants, with ADHD individuals being at the highest risk of abusing or diverting their stimulant prescriptions. Data from the Care Quality Commission (2013) reveals that between 16 and 29 per cent of students who are prescribed stimulants report diverting their prescriptions. Between 5 and 9 per cent of primary and high school children and between 5 and 35 per cent of college students have used non-prescribed stimulants. Most often their motivation is to concentrate, improve alertness, get high, or to experiment. Stimulant medications may be resold by patients as recreational drugs, and Methylphenidate is used as a study aid by some students without ADHD.

Evidence also exists of possible differences of race and ethnicity in the prevalence of ADHD. The prevalence of ADHD dramatically varies across cultures despite the fact that the same methodology has been used. Is this due to different perceptions of what qualifies as disruptive behaviour, inattention and hyperactivity? Does the distribution of ADHD diagnosis fall along socio-economic lines, according to the amount of wealth within a neighbourhood, and may assist in the establishment of a misdiagnosis of ADHD? Does the application of national, general guidelines to localised and specific contexts, such as where referral is unavailable, CAMH resources are lacking, increase the risk of a misdiagnosis of ADHD?

What are the features of ADHD to look out for?

Usually there need to be problems both at home and school serious enough to affect family functioning or academic achievement. The symptoms must have started before the age of seven and cannot be accounted for by depression or anxiety. Specific features to consider when assessing for a full diagnosis of ADHD are:

Six or more of the following:

- Failure to pay close attention to detail, makes frequent mistakes.

- Difficulty in concentrating on tasks or play activities.

- Failure to listen when spoken to directly.

- Failure to follow through on instructions or finish tasks.

- Lack of organisation.

- Reluctance to start tasks that require concentration.

- Loses items necessary to complete tasks.

- Distracted by irrelevant activity.

- Forgetful in daily activities.

Chapter 6: What are the current issues challenging young people?

125

Three or more of the following:

- Fidgets.

- Cannot remain seated.

- Inappropriate running or climbing.

- Noisy.

- Being constantly active.

One or more of the following:

- Blurts out answers before a question is completed.

- Failure to wait in turn.

- Interrupts or intrudes on others' conversations or games.

- Talks constantly.

Staff should offer parents or carers of pre-school children with ADHD a referral to a parent-training/education programme as the first-line treatment if the parents or carers have not already attended such a programme or the programme has had a limited effect. Teachers who have received training about ADHD and its management could provide behavioural interventions in the classroom to help children and young people with ADHD.

If the child or young person with ADHD has moderate levels of impairment, the parents or carers should be offered referral to a group parent-training/education programme, either on its own or together with a group treatment programme (CBT and/or social skills training) for the child or young person. In school-age children and young people with severe ADHD, drug treatment should be offered as the first-line treatment. Parents should also be offered a group-based parent-training/education programme. Drug treatment for children and young people with ADHD should always form part of a comprehensive treatment plan that includes psychological, behavioural and educational advice and interventions.

If the child or young person's behavioural and/or attention problems suggestive of ADHD are having an adverse impact on their development or family life, social workers should consider a period of watchful waiting of up to 10 weeks and offer parents/ carers a referral to a parent-training/education programme. If the behavioural and/ or attention problems persist with at least moderate impairment, the child or young person should be referred to a child psychiatrist, paediatrician or specialist ADHD CAMHS for assessment.

Group-based parent-training/education programmes are usually the first-line treatment for parents and carers of children and young people of school age with ADHD and moderate impairment. This may also include group psychological treatment CBT and/or social skills training for the younger child. For older age groups, individual psychological treatment may be more acceptable if group behavioural or psychological approaches have not been effective, or have been refused.

Is ADHD over-diagnosed?

Issues with co-morbidity are a possible explanation in favour of the argument of over-diagnosis. In medicine, co-morbidity is the presence of one or more additional diseases or disorders co-occurring with (that is, concomitant or concurrent with) a primary disease or disorder. As many as 75 per cent of diagnosed children with ADHD meet criteria for some other psychiatric diagnosis (Banaschewski et al, 2015). Among children diagnosed with ADHD, about 25 to 30 per cent have anxiety disorders, 9 to 32 per cent have depression, 45 to 84 per cent have oppositional defiant disorder, and 44 to 55 per cent of adolescents have conduct disorder. Learning disorders are found in 20 to 40 per cent of children with ADHD.

Another possible explanation for over-diagnosis of ADHD is the relative-age effect, which applies to children of both sexes. Younger children are more likely to be inappropriately diagnosed with ADHD and treated with prescription medication than their older peers in the same school year. Children who are almost a year younger tend to appear more immature than their classmates, which influences both their academic and athletic performance.

Gender differences

Research on gender differences from Banaschewski et al (2015) also reveals an argument for under-diagnosis of ADHD among girls. The ratio for male-to-female is four to one with 92 per cent of girls with ADHD receiving a primarily inattentive subtype diagnosis. This difference in gender can be explained, for the majority, by the different ways in which boys and girls express symptoms of this particular disorder. Typically, females with ADHD exhibit less disruptive behaviours and more internalising behaviours. Girls tend to show fewer behavioural problems, show fewer aggressive behaviours, are less impulsive, and are less hyperactive than boys diagnosed with ADHD.

Chapter 6: What are the current issues challenging young people?

127

These patterns of behaviour are less likely to disrupt the classroom or home setting, therefore allowing parents and teachers to easily overlook or neglect the presence of a potential problem. The current diagnostic criteria appear to be more geared towards males than females, and the ADHD characteristics of men have been over-represented.

This leaves many women and girls with ADHD neglected. Studies have shown that girls with ADHD, especially those with signs of impulsivity, were three to four times more likely to attempt suicide when compared with female controls. Additionally, these girls were two to three times more likely to engage in self-harming behaviours.

Refugee and asylum seekers

Refugee and asylum-seeking children are a new community and are among the most disadvantaged ethnic minority group for whom socially inclusive CAMH practice is essential. Some are unaccompanied, and many severely affected by extreme circumstances might include those witnessing the murder of parents or kin, dislocation from school and community, and severing of important friendships. Race hate is becoming an everyday experience. Lack of extended family support, loss of home and prolonged insecurity add to their sense of vulnerability. These experiences can trigger symptoms of post-traumatic stress disorder and a variety of mental health problems.

Parents' coping strategies and overall resilience can be diminished in these trying circumstances, disrupting the self-regulatory patterns of comfort and family support usually available at times of stress. Involvement needs to take a broad holistic and integrated approach to intervention and not overlook the need for careful assessment of mental health problems developing in adults and children, while responding to practical demands. If these are not tackled promptly, these young people may go on to develop serious and persistent difficulties which are harder, and more costly, to resolve in the long term.

The scale of the level of need can be gauged by considering that the number of applications for asylum in the UK from unaccompanied under 18s almost trebled in recent years so that over the past four years, there have been just over 11,315 applications by asylum-seeking children less than 18 years old in the UK. The number of applications from unaccompanied children, excluding dependants, was 3,043 in 2015, a 56 per cent increase compared with 2014. The largest number of applications from unaccompanied asylum-seeking children in 2018 were from Sudan, Eritrea and Vietnam (Refugee Council, 2018).

Further evidence shows that many of these young people were accommodated or placed in detention centres and receiving a worse service than other children in need.

Very little research has been done to ascertain the psychological needs of this group of children. However, there is some evidence of the symptoms of post-traumatic stress disorder being present before they then experience the racist and xenophobic abuse of individuals and institutions incapable of demonstrating humanitarian concern for their plight. This combination can shatter the most psychologically robust personality. It has been estimated that serious mental health disorders may be present in 40 to 50 per cent of young refugees (Refugee Council, 2018).

✒ Activity 6.3 Case illustration

A family of Syrian asylum seekers fled the country recently. The father, Mohammad, had worked in the petroleum industry. Mohammad claims he was tortured and had death threats made against his wife and three children who are of Kurdish origin. The children are all under eight years of age and his wife Shirez is a nursery teacher. Some of the children speak very little English. The family have been relocated to a small town where there are very few Syrians, or any families from Middle Eastern countries. The local housing department have referred the family to your office following reports of racist attacks in the bed and breakfast hostel where they have been housed in emergency accommodation. A teacher has called your team four times in the past fortnight expressing concern about one of the male children who is 7 years old, speaks English well but is wetting and soiling himself in class, provoking bullying from other children.

💬 Commentary

Your first task is to begin the process of assessment by constructing a visual map of all the people, agencies and services connected to this family. You will find it helpful to then make contact with as many as you can within a realistic timescale to start to plan your response. This information-gathering exercise will enable you to begin to evaluate the different agendas and perceptions of other staff working with or concerned with the family. Your priority is to establish meaningful contact with the family and gain factual evidence of racist incidents for possible criminal prosecution against the perpetrators, as well as offering a caring, sympathetic relationship. Bear in mind that the family are likely to be highly suspicious of your motives and will require a lot of genuine evidence that they should trust you. Their naturally defensive behaviour may come across as hostile or uncommunicative and you need to deal with this in a non-confrontational manner.

A translator or interpreter should accompany you having been fully briefed beforehand about your task, the different roles each of you holds, and to assess their suitability for this particular task. Do not assume that every interpreter is the same, and try to evaluate their beliefs or attitudes and whether there may be ethnic or religious

Chapter 6: What are the current issues challenging young people?

129

differences between them and the family. For a variety of reasons they might be inappropriate for this task despite having the right language skills. Strict translation of words and terms will be unhelpful; therefore, time needs to be spent on the interpretation of the interpretation. Right from the start you can better engage with the family by:

- enabling everyone to have their say;

- using sensitive questioning to enable expression of feelings;

- reinforcing the integrity of the family system;

- noting patterns of communication and structure.

Having established a helping relationship, a holistic perspective enables you to locate the family system within a wider system of agencies, resources and a local environment that is generally hostile. Your networking skills can mobilise the statutory agencies to provide what is required to attend to the immediate areas of concern and clarify roles and responsibilities. A case conference or network meeting can put this on a formal basis with an action checklist for future reference to monitor the plan. One option may be to plan some family sessions together with a colleague from another agency such as Health or Education.

This could combine assessment and intervention work to ascertain medium-term needs while using therapeutic skills to help the family establish their equilibrium. The key is to enable them to re-establish their particular coping mechanisms and ways of dealing with stress, rather than trying to impose an artificial solution. Maintaining a systems-wide perspective can help you evaluate the factors and elements building up to form a contemporary picture of their context. Working with them as a family and demonstrating simple things like reliability and consistency will provide them with an emotional anchor – a secure-enough base to begin to manage themselves in due course.

The 7 year-old child is demonstrating symptoms of severe trauma and anxiety and needs a referral to a specialist CAMHS team, but there will inevitably be a waiting list for treatment so you can arrange individual sessions involving play, drawing, puppets, games, etc, to engage him. Once a trusting relationship is established you can encourage him to talk about his fears and worries. You may feel you are out of your depth but often simple things can make a big impact, and you should ensure you have access to supervision/guidance from the CAMHS team if you feel concerned, while the child waits for an appointment.

Lesbian, gay, bisexual and transgender youth

The way in which homosexuality and sexual orientation is perceived by children and young people can be considerably influenced by social and media representations. For some young people struggling with their identity during developmental transitions, this social context can serve to enhance feelings of shame or encourage a sense of pride. Without doubt however, for some this context can result in mental health problems.

Very high levels of suicide among young males and the burgeoning literature on the widely reported crisis of identity among young men is sometimes explained as a result of being challenged by years of feminist critiques of patriarchal society and gender abuse of power. Workers need to consider very carefully and understand how children and young people construct and internalise concepts of gender and sexuality. The invisibility of lesbian and gay role models or thoughtful discussion in social contexts conspire to construct a sense of danger and shame as adolescents experiment and explore different aspects of their sexuality.

An interesting research study (Walker, 2016) explored the use of homophobic terms by boys and young men and the meanings invoked when they use them in order to find evidence that might help explain masculinity and adult sexual identity formation in later years. The study found that homophobic terms come into currency in primary school but usually with little connection with sexual connotations. The effect seems to be that early homophobic experiences provide an important reference point for boys and young men comprehending forthcoming sexual identity formation. A progressive approach in this area demands a balanced and open mind.

Evidence shows that teachers report high levels of homophobic, biphobic and transphobic bullying among schoolchildren. Most teachers are not sure how to tackle this issue and a majority have not had specific training to equip them to deal with it or how to teach these subjects. One in five young people have missed school due to this bullying and are vulnerable to developing mental health problems because of bullying, stigma and family attitudes. A significant number have self-harmed or attempted suicide.

✎ Activity 6.4

🔦 Discuss this issue with a colleague and be honest about any prejudice or assumptions you both carry about sexuality.

🔦 Consider how you might increase your awareness and enable a young person you are working with to be open about any of these issues underlying their mental health problems.

☐ Commentary

It's important not to make assumptions about who is lesbian, gay, bisexual or transgender (LGBT). Let a young person use the words of their choice to describe their sexual orientation or gender identity and remember that every young person will express who they are in their own way. When a young person comes out as lesbian, gay, bisexual or transgender, listen, offer reassurance and talk to them about how they'd like to proceed. Parents/carers need to know that LGBT issues are covered in school. Don't discuss a young person's sexual orientation or gender identity with parents/carers without the young person's permission. Work with supportive parents/carers to ensure the best support for a young person and know where to signpost should parents/carers want information, advice or support. Teachers can take a whole-school approach to tackling homophobic, biphobic and transphobic bullying and language and challenge gender stereotypes from an early age. It will be helpful to find out what's running in the local community and support young people to set up diversity or peer support groups in school. Providing LGBT young people with relevant information and resources so they are able to make safe choices is crucial. You can help young people stay safe online and when out and about. Make sure young people know their rights and how to report discrimination. Ensure young people know how they can access counselling and mental health services. LGBT people and experiences should be reflected in the school curriculum, including in sex and relationships education. There are a range of books with LGBT characters and different families that can now be accessed.

What are the key issues in supporting LGBT young people?

• You do not need to be an expert in LGBT young people's lives – using a person-centred approach will ensure that you will understand their experience and enable you to provide effective support.

• It is important to involve young people in decisions that affect their lives. If you are working directly with an LGBT young person, take time to listen to their experiences and make decisions that take their views into consideration.

• LGBT young people can receive negative messages regarding their identities and who they are. It is therefore important to be non-judgemental in your approach and provide positive and supportive messages regarding their feelings, thoughts and identities.

• Confidentiality is of the utmost importance to LGBT young people. You will have to share issues relating to child protection or vulnerable adults at risk; however, issues pertaining to sexual orientation or gender identity alone are not justification to share information.

Transgender children

National media are increasingly presenting stories of a group of young transgender children (those who persistently, insistently, and consistently identify as the gender identity that is the opposite of their natal sex). A large number of these children have socially transitioned; they are being raised and are presenting to others as their gender identity rather than their natal sex, a reversible non-medical intervention that involves changing the pronouns used to describe a child, as well as his or her name and typically hair length and clothing.

These stories have sparked an international debate about whether parents of young transgender children should support their children's desire to live presenting as their gender identity. Despite considerable and heated discussion on the topic, and despite these children's increasing appearance at gender clinics, there is little research on the mental health of transgender children who have socially transitioned, forcing workers to make recommendations to parents without any systematic, empirical investigations of mental health among socially transitioned children.

Most studies of mental health among transgender people have examined adolescents and adults. These studies consistently report dramatically elevated rates of anxiety, depression and suicidality among transgender people. These are likely the result of years of prejudice, discrimination and stigma; conflict between one's appearance and stated identity; and general rejection by people in their social environments, including their families. There is now growing evidence that social support is linked to better mental health outcomes among transgender adolescents. Social transitions in children, a form of affirmation and support by a prepubescent child's parents, could be associated with good mental health outcomes in transgender children.

How to support transgender children

The following principles are based on good practice recommendations and the UN Convention of the Rights of the Child (UNCRC).

• Transgender young people should be protected from discrimination, harm and abuse.

• Expressing gender is a healthy part of growing up. It is unethical to force a young person to express their gender in a particular way.

• If a transgender young person needs support, they should get this as soon as possible and at a pace which is right for them.

- Being transgender is one aspect of a young person's life; it is important to recognise they may have other support needs.

- Transgender young people should be involved in all decisions affecting them, understand any action which is taken and why; and be at the centre of any decision-making.

- Wherever possible, staff should respect a transgender young person's right to privacy. Being transgender is not a child protection or well-being concern.

Summary of key points

- Relative child poverty in the UK is projected to rise between 2010 and 2020 from 17.5 per cent to 23.5 per cent, or over 1 million children. One-quarter of all rape victims are children and 75 per cent of sexually abused children do not tell anyone at the time. Each year about 30,000 children are on child protection registers. Recorded offences of gross indecency with a child more than doubled from 1985 to 2010, and last year there were 46,352 offences but convictions against perpetrators actually fell from 42 per cent to 19 per cent.

- Self-harm is an increasing problem. Some young people may self-harm just once or twice. For others it can become a habitual response to any overwhelming situation. It is important that the issue is addressed immediately, and assessment is the gateway to understanding and future management. It is rare for self-harming behaviour to exist in isolation.

- Mental health problems result from cyberbullying as a consequence of the way an individual reacts to the chronic stress of being consistently involved in predictable, aggressive and humiliating situations. Apart from anxiety and depression, other symptoms include: not sleeping well, bed wetting, feeling sad, experiencing headaches and having tummy aches. It has been estimated that between 15 and 25 young victims of cyberbullying commit suicide each year in the UK.

- Multicultural counselling and therapy help a young person develop a greater awareness about themselves in relation to their different family and social contexts. This results in support that is contextual in orientation and which is able to respectfully draw on traditional methods of healing with a spiritual or religious dimension from many cultures.

★ Traditional binary definitions of sexuality are diminishing among growing numbers of young people. It is important to involve young people in decisions that affect their lives. If you are working directly with an LGBT young person, take time to listen to their experiences and make decisions that take their views into consideration.

Further reading

Bartram, F (2017) *An Introduction to Supporting LGBT Young People: A Guide for Schools*. London: Stonewall Education.

Bhugra, D, Craig, T and Bhui, K (2010) *Mental Health of Refugees and Asylum Seekers*. Oxford: Oxford University Press.

Hinduja, S and Patchin, J (2014) *Bullying Beyond the Schoolyard: Preventing and Responding to Cyberbullying*. Thousand Oaks, CA: Sage.

Saint-Exupery, A (2015) *The Little Prince*. New York: Seaburn Books.

Walker, S (2012) *Responding to Self-Harm in Children and Adolescents*. London: Jessica Kingsley.

Williamson, L (2016) *The Art of Being Normal*. Oxford: David Fickling Books.

✋ Internet resources

✋ Refugee and asylum seekers: **www.asylumaid.org.uk**

✋ Rethink Mental Illness: **www.rethink.org**

✋ Self-harm: **www.selfharm.co.uk**

Chapter 6: What are the current issues challenging young people?

135

Chapter 7: How to promote young people's rights and mental health

Introduction

The promotion of young people's rights in the context of their mental health problems is as important as it is complex. In 1989 the United Nations (UN) General Assembly adopted a landmark – the Convention on the Rights of the Child (CRC) (Unicef, 1989). The Convention recognised that children are human beings and more than just *'passive objects of care and charity'* who are entitled to the enjoyment of a distinct set of rights in accordance with their specific needs. The CRC provides clear guidance and a monitoring framework against which to evaluate progress towards the realisation of children's right to health:

- from child mortality;

- combating disease and malnutrition;

- preventing violence and injury;

- ensuring rehabilitation and support for children with disabilities;

- abolishing traditional practices that harm children such as early enforced marriage and female genital mutilation.

The United Kingdom ratified the Convention in 1991, with several declarations and reservations, and made its first report to the Committee on the Rights of the Child in January 1995. Concerns raised by the Committee about British children included the growth in child poverty and inequality, the extent of violence towards children, the use of custody for young offenders, the low age of criminal responsibility, and the lack of opportunities for children and young people to express views. The 2002 report of the Committee expressed similar concerns, including the welfare of children in custody, unequal treatment of asylum seekers, and the negative impact of poverty on children's rights. In September 2008, the UK government decided to withdraw its reservations and agree to the Convention in these respects.

Thanks to the context of the CRC, there is a growing emphasis on children's rights and the importance of enabling children and young people to influence decisions about their own health and social welfare. There is also emphasis on developing innovative methods of eliciting their views and enabling young people to identify their own agenda as far as possible, rather than responding to an adult-imposed one.

Why is empowering young people important?

Focusing on the organisation and delivery of child and adolescent mental health services, as well as managing the challenges in multi-disciplinary working and training, runs the risk of neglecting young people's perceptions and experiences. The evidence of adult client/patient/service user consultation, over changes in service provision in health and social care, is limited. For children's services in general, it is unusual. Children and young people's perspectives have rarely been explored in relation to the help they are offered towards their mental health difficulties. As a professional or parent, it is critical that you work hard to seize every opportunity to enable a troubled young person to express their wishes and feelings about the kind of support they want.

Key legal and policy guidelines

Children's rights are becoming embedded in legal and policy frameworks around child and adolescent mental health services. The following are the key legal and policy context and guidelines within which assessment and intervention take place. Whatever agency you work in, or whether you are a parent or young person, it is helpful to know the legal and policy boundaries within which helping activity takes place. Knowing the limits to your work and having an understanding of legal rights and responsibilities are critical.

Government policies

The 2010–15 Coalition government committed to improving mental health for children and young people, as part of their commitment to achieving 'parity of esteem' between physical and mental health, and to improving the lives of children and young people. The 2011 mental health strategy *No Health Without Mental Health* pledged to provide early support for mental health problems, and the former Deputy Prime Minister's 2014 strategy *Closing the Gap: priorities for essential change in mental health* included actions such as improving access to psychological therapies for children and young people. The Department of Health and NHS England established a Children and Young People's Mental Health and Wellbeing Taskforce which reported in March 2015: *Future in Mind*, and set out ambitions for improving care over the next five years.

The 2015–17 government announced new funding for mental health, including specific investment in perinatal services and eating disorder services for teenagers. Additionally, the 2015 government committed to implementing the recommendations made in *The Five Year Forward View for Mental Health* (February 2016), including specific objectives to improve treatment for children and young people by 2020–1. The *Policing and Crime Act 2017* legislates to end the practice of children and young people being kept in police cells as a 'place of safety' while they await mental health assessment or treatment.

As a recent joint report from the Health and Education Select Committee's notes, schools have a front-line role in children and young people's mental health. There has been a drive to improve the provision of mental health support in schools, and to foster closer working between the health and education systems. In June 2014, the Department for Education published guidance for schools on identifying and supporting pupils who may have mental health problems. In March 2015, the Department for Education provided schools with practical, evidence-based advice on how to deliver high-quality school-based counselling, and guidance on teaching about mental health problems.

The government has said that schools are encouraged to teach about mental health in personal, social and health education (PSHE) and that the PSHE association, with government funding, has produced a guide on preparing to teach about mental health and emotional well-being. Since then, the PSHE association has also published a programme of study, which includes mental health at Key Stages 4 and 5 and social media at Key Stages 2 to 5. The government is considering making PSHE a statutory requirement. Following a speech by the Prime Minister on transforming mental health support, a Green Paper on children and young people's mental health was published in December 2017, which proposed improving mental health support in schools and colleges, and trialling a four-week waiting-time standard for access to mental health treatment. However, data from Freedom of Information requests by the British Medical Association show that many Clinical Commissioning Groups are not increasing their spending on CAMHS. In a 2017 BMA survey of CAMHS professionals, 91 per cent of respondents felt that CAMHS is poorly funded, and 58 per cent felt that changes to CAMHS funding levels had made them less able to do their job (Royal College of GPs, 2017).

The legal framework

The legal framework for child and adolescent mental health encompasses a wide spectrum of social policy including juvenile justice, mental health, education, and children and family legislation. An important point is that the term *mental illness* is not defined in law relating to children and young people. The variety of legal frameworks affecting them provide the context for work undertaken by a number of parents, teachers and health and social care staff concerned about children and young people whose behaviour is described as disturbed or disturbing. Of particular interest in the context of empowering practice are the issues of consent and confidentiality. The

Children's Legal Centre has drawn attention to a number of issues regarding the rights of children and young people who might have contact with agencies on the basis of their mental health problems.

• Lack of knowledge and implementation of legal rights for children and young people to control their own medical treatment, and a general lack of rights to self-determination.

• Discrimination against children and young people on the grounds of disability, race, culture, colour, language, religion, gender and sexuality, which can lead to categorisation as mentally ill and subsequent intervention and detention.

• Unnecessary and in some cases unlawful restriction of liberty and inadequate safeguards in mental health and other legislation for children and young people.

• Inadequate assessment and corresponding lack of care, treatment and education in the criminal justice system.

• Use of drugs for containment rather than treatment purposes in the community, schools and in other institutions, combined with a lack of knowledge of consent procedures.

• Placement of children on adult wards in psychiatric hospitals.

• Lack of clear ethical guidelines for extreme situations such as force-feedings in cases of anorexia, care of suicide-risk young people, and care of HIV-positive or AIDS patients.

The organisational complexity

Children with mental health problems may move between four overlapping systems: criminal justice, social services, education and the health service. Children are not always helped by the appropriate service since this often depends on the resources available in the area at the time. It also depends on how different professional staff may perceive the behaviour of a particular child, and the vocabulary used by the service in which they work. A youth offending team member may talk about a young person engaged in anti-social activity, a teacher about poor concentration and aggressive behaviour, and a social worker may perceive a needy, anxious, abused child. All are describing the same child.

✎ Activity 7.1 Case illustration

At a multi-agency meeting you find yourself considering the case of a young female, 14 years of age with a history of self-harm and school refusal. She is described by her parents as 'moody' and 'uncommunicative'. The school nurse noticed recent parallel cut marks on her arm when she administered a year-wide immunisation. The girl did not respond to questions about the marks. The police have been involved with her in the past due to incidents of shoplifting and gang-related alcohol abuse. The teacher reports that she has a poor attendance record and is hard working but low on ability when she does attend lessons. As far as social services are concerned, there has been sporadic contact with the family over the past few years with one younger brother sustaining one incident of non-accidental injury. There are four other children in the household and the father has a history of alcoholism and domestic violence.

➤ Prepare an action plan for a multi-agency team meeting, with alternatives.
➤ Work out what your role might be.
➤ Anticipate what options other professionals are going to suggest.
➤ How are you going to demonstrate a children's rights model of practice?

💬 Commentary

The multi-agency meeting is a critical opportunity to assess the level of need in this situation and what resources and responses are available and appropriate. These include family and wider community resources as well as personal resources and potential within the young person. The pathway of a child into the formal state systems is crucial because the consequences for subsequent intervention can either exacerbate the behaviour or help to reduce it. Discuss your answers to the above questions with a mentor or supervisor, and undertake research to examine the evidence base on similar situations. Comprehensive, flexible preparation can maximise the potential for the optimum response. Table 7.1 illustrates schematically potential agency responses to the same presenting problem. In this illustration, the young person has been labelled as aggressive.

The Crime and Disorder Act 1998 and the Special Educational Needs and Disability Act 2001 provide the legislative framework for youth justice and children with special educational needs. In both cases, children and young people with mental health problems may find they are being inappropriately dealt with under these Acts. The Mental Health Act 1983, the Children Act 1989 and the Human Rights Act 1998 are currently the three significant pieces of legislation providing the context for practice in child and adolescent mental health.

Table 7.1 Agency responses to the same presenting problem

Juvenile justice	Social services	Education	Psychiatry
Aggressive	Aggressive	Aggressive	Aggressive
Referral to police: decision to charge ↓	Referral to social services ↓	Referral to education department ↓	Referral to child psychiatrist ↓
Pre-sentence report completed ↓	Social work assessment conducted ↓	Educational psychology assessment ↓	Psychiatric assessment ↓
Sentenced to custody ↓	Decision to accommodate ↓	Placed in residential school ↓	Admitted to regional in-patient unit ↓
Labelled as *young offender*	Labelled as *beyond parental control*	Labelled as *having learning difficulty*	Labelled as *mentally ill*

Mental Health Act 1983

In 2017, 47 children were detained under the Mental Health Act and placed in unsuitable adult psychiatric establishments, according to official government statistics (Office for National Statistics, 2017). Campaigners, parents and CAMH professionals have repeatedly expressed concern about the safety of children in adult psychiatric wards. The Mental Health Act 1983 is a piece of legislation designed mainly for adults with mental health problems and, among other things, sets the framework for the assessment and potential compulsory admission of patients to hospital. The majority of children in psychiatric hospitals or units are informal patients. They do not have the same access to safeguards available to adult patients detained under the Mental Health Act 1983.

Children under 16 are frequently admitted by their parents even though they may not have wanted to be admitted. This is *de facto* detention. The number of children admitted to NHS psychiatric units designed for young people has risen in recent years. In 1995, 4,891 children and young people under the age of 19 were referred in England. By 2000 the number had risen to 5,788, an increase of 18 per cent. In 2013, there were nearly 8,000 young people referred for in-patient admission (Walker, 2016). This is a worrying trend, which is also reflected in the adult statistics for compulsory admissions. Health and social care policy is meant to be shifting resources away from institutional-based provision to community care, but in the context of troubled young people the reverse appears to be the case.

Parts 2 and 3 of the Mental Health Act 1983 provide for compulsory admission and continued detention where a child or young person is deemed to have, or is suspected of having, a mental disorder. The mental disorder must be specified as mental illness, psychopathic disorder, learning disability, or severe mental impairment. Learning disability is not stated as such in the Act, and as with psychopathic disorder, it must be associated with abnormally aggressive or seriously irresponsible conduct. Full assessment and treatment orders under Sections 2 and 3 require an application to be made by the nearest relative or an Approved Mental Health Professional under the 2007 Mental Health Act, together with medical recommendation by two doctors. Approved Mental Health Professionals have a critical role in safeguarding the rights of children and young people at these rare and acute episodes in their lives. The sections of the Mental Health Act 1983 most likely to be used with children and young people are:

> **Section 2:** for assessment for possible admission for up to 28 days.

> **Section 4:** for an emergency assessment for up to 72 hours' admission.

> **Section 5 (2):** for emergency detention by one doctor for up to 72 hours.

> **Section 5 (4):** for emergency six-hour detention when no doctor or social worker is available.

> **Section 3:** for in-patient treatment for a treatable disorder for up to six months.

Why is consent an important factor?

Defining the capacity of a child to make her or his own decisions and consent to intervention is not easy, especially in the area of child mental health. The concept of *Gillick competent* arose following a landmark ruling in 1985 in the House of Lords (3 All E.R. 402, 1985). That ruling held that competent children under 16 years of age can consent to and refuse advice and treatment from a doctor. Since then, further court cases have modified the Gillick principle so that if either the child or any person with parental responsibility gives consent to treatment, doctors can proceed, even if one or more of these people, including the child, disagree. The preferred term now is *Fraser competent* after the presiding judge in those later cases.

The concept of *competent* refers to a child having the capacity to understand the nature, terms and consequences of the proposed treatment, or the consequences of refusing such treatment, free from pressure to comply. In practice, children are considered to be lacking in capacity to consent although this could be as a result of underestimating children's intelligence, or more likely reflect an inability to communicate effectively with them. Courts have consistently held that children do not have sufficient understanding of death – hence the force-feeding of anorexics and blood transfusions of Jehovah's Witnesses.

Court of Appeal decisions have since overturned the principle that Fraser-competent children can refuse treatment. Such cases involved extreme and life-threatening situations involving anorexia, blood transfusion, and severely disturbed behaviour. Importantly, the courts have indicated that any person with parental responsibility can in certain circumstances override the refusal of a Fraser-competent child. This means that children under a care order or accommodated by the local authority, even if considered not to have the capacity to consent, still retain the right to be consulted about the proposed treatment. If a child is accommodated, a social worker should always obtain the parents' consent since they retain full parental responsibility. If the child is under a care order, the parents share parental responsibility with the local authority. Good practice requires the social worker in these situations to negotiate with parents about who should give consent and ensure that all views are recorded in the care plan.

Confidentiality

Children and young people require the help and advice of a wide variety of sources at times of stress and unhappiness in their lives. There are voluntary, statutory and private agencies as well as relatives or friends who they find easier to approach than parents. They may want to talk in confidence about worrying feelings or behaviour. The legal position in these circumstances is confused, with agencies and professional groups such as counsellors or psychotherapists relying on voluntary codes of practice guidance. A difficult dilemma frequently arises when children are considering whether a helping service is acceptable while the staff are required to disclose information to others in certain situations, for example where child protection concerns are aroused.

How can you ensure a child is informed and included in the process?

The agency policies should be accessible to children and clearly state the limits to confidentiality. But in doing so, many practitioners know they could be discouraging the sharing of important feelings and information. Staff know only too well the importance of establishing trust and confidence in vulnerable young people and constantly have to tread the line between facilitating sensitive communication and selecting what needs to be passed on to parents, colleagues or to third parties. Ideally, where disclosure needs to be made against a young person's wishes it is good practice to inform the young person in advance and give her or him the chance to disclose the information first.

The Data Protection Act 2018 and the Access to Personal Files Act 1987 give individuals the right to see information about them, with some limitations. Children *of sufficient understanding* have the right of access except in certain circumstances. These are particularly relevant:

• where disclosure would be likely to cause serious harm to the child's physical or mental health;

• where the information would disclose the identity of another person;

• where the information is contained within a court report;

• where the information is restricted or prohibited from disclosure in adoption cases;

• where the information is a statement of special education needs made under the Education Act 1981.

Updates to the Mental Health Act 1983 came into force in 2008 with the Mental Health Act 2007. These included: a single definition of mental disorder; changing the criteria for detention by abolishing the Treatability Test and introducing a new Appropriate Treatment Test. Importantly, changes also included a directive to ensure that age-appropriate services are available for any young person aged under 18 admitted to hospital. Young people now have the ability to apply to court to change their nearest relative, and they are ensured the right to an advocacy service when under compulsion.

Importantly, the UK at long last signed up in full to the United Nations Convention on the Rights of the Child. The UK government had maintained an opt out since 1991, due to the Conservative government's unease about granting better protections to children in the context of a debate about parental rights and the use of smacking and physical chastisement, which meant they did not fully accept responsibilities to asylum-seeking children to appropriate protection and assistance. Now asylum-seeking children have the same protection and access to services as other children, although such children are still subject to inhumane detention and financial constraints which adversely affect their mental health.

Children Act 1989

A child who is suffering with mental health problems may behave in ways that stretch their parents' or carers' capacity to cope, which can result in the potential for significant harm. On the other hand, a child who is being abused or neglected may come to the attention of professionals concerned initially about their mental health. The interactive nature of mental health and child abuse presents a considerable challenge for workers tasked with conducting assessment work in child and family contexts. In terms of the Children Act, social workers operate within deceptively clear guidelines. In practice however, the provisions within the Act and subsequent practice guidelines have sought to bring simplicity to what are inevitably highly complex situations. The duties under the terms of the Children Act are straightforward and underpinned by the following principles.

- The welfare of the child is paramount.

- Children should be brought up and cared for within their own families wherever possible.

- Children should be safe and protected by effective interventions if at risk.

- Courts should avoid delay and only make an order if this is better than not making an order.

- Children should be kept informed about what happens to them and involved in decisions made about them.

- Parents continue to have parental responsibility for their children even when their children are no longer living with them.

The shift in emphasis heralded by the Children Act from investigative child protection to needs-led assessment for family support services is particularly significant for social workers engaged in work involving children's mental health. There is a specific legal requirement under the Act that different authorities and agencies work together to provide family support services with better liaison and a corporate approach.

Together with the four-tier integrated child and adolescent mental health services structure, the framework is there to achieve better co-ordination and effectiveness of services to help any family with a child who has a mental health problem. This is made clear under the terms of Section 17 of the Children Act that lays a duty on local authorities to provide services for children in need. The definition of *in need* has three elements:

- the child is unlikely to achieve or maintain, or to have the opportunity of achieving or maintaining, a reasonable standard of health or development without the provision for the child of services by a local authority; or

- the child's health or development is likely to be significantly impaired, or further impaired, without provision for the child of such services; or

- the child is disabled.

How is disability defined?

The Act further defines disability as including children suffering from mental disorder of any kind. In relation to the first two parts of the definition, health or development is defined to cover physical, intellectual, emotional, social or behavioural development and physical or mental health. These concepts are open to interpretation of what is meant by a *'reasonable standard of health and development'*, as well as the predictive implications for children having the *'opportunity'* of achieving or maintaining it. However, it is reasonable to include the following groups of children within this part of the definition of *in need* and to argue the case for preventive support where there is a risk of children developing mental health problems:

- children living in poverty;

- homeless children;

- children suffering the effects of racism;

- young carers;

- delinquent children;

- children separated from parent(s).

Some children from these groups may be truanting from school, getting involved in criminal activities, or have behaviour problems at school and/or home. Agency responses will tend to address the presenting problem and try an intervention to apparently address it. Assessment of the needs of individual children and families is often cursory, deficit-oriented and static. The Common Assessment Framework offers the opportunity for social workers – in collaboration with other professionals – to conduct more positive, comprehensive assessments that permit the mental health needs of children and adolescents to be illuminated.

✎ Activity 7.2

🔸 At your next team/student group meeting, present a case in which the assessment of a child or young person raised issues about whether the child was 'in need' as defined in the Children Act 1989.

🔸 Ask the group to consider the information available and then to make an individual judgement.

🔸 Compare and contrast the different responses and discuss.

💬 Commentary

Section 47 of the Children Act gives the local authority a duty to investigate where they suspect a child is suffering or is likely to suffer significant harm. Guidance suggests the purpose of such an investigation is to establish facts, decide if there are grounds for concern, identify risk, and decide protective action. The problem with child and adolescent mental health problems is that this guidance assumes certainty within a time-limited assessment period. The nature of emotional and behavioural difficulties is their often hidden quality combined with the child's own reluctance to acknowledge them.

The interpretation of a child or young person's emotional or behavioural state is usually decided by a child and adolescent psychiatrist who may be brought into a Section 43 child assessment order that has been sought following parental lack of co-operation. The social worker in situations like this, and in full care proceedings, has a crucial role in balancing the need to protect the child with the future consequences on them and their family of oppressive investigations and interventions.

In cases where the child's competence to consent to treatment, or capacity to express their wishes and feelings, is impaired, it is likely that the Children Act 1989 should be used in preference to the Mental Health Act 1983. The Children Act does not carry the same stigma and consequences of the Mental Health Act, and it provides for a children's guardian to consider all the factors and act as an independent advocate in legal proceedings. The Children Act aimed to consolidate a number of childcare reforms and provide a response to the evidence of failure in children's services that had been mounting in the 1980s.

The role of the advocate

Prior to the Children Act 1989, professional practice was perceived as intrusive, legalistic and biased towards child protection investigation. The new Act tried to redress the balance towards identifying needs and providing support to parents to prevent harm or neglect of children and young people. Contemporary debate about the Children Act is still concerned with how to translate the widely endorsed principles of the legislation into practical help for child welfare service users and providers. In the context of child and adolescent mental health, this requires workers to optimise professional knowledge, skills and values in a very complex area of practice.

One of the distinctive roles for all workers in this context is that of advocate. This may seem contradictory in cases where the local authority is acting in the child's best interests, but in terms of establishing trust, respect and relationship building, supporting a complaint has benefit for staff involved in CAMHS. Section 26 of the Children Act provides for a complaints procedure through which children and young people can appeal against decisions reached by social workers. There are informal and formal stages to the procedure with an expectation that an independent person is included at the formal stages. When these procedures have been exhausted, a judicial review can be applied for within three months of the decision being appealed against. The three grounds for succeeding with judicial review are:

- **ultra vires:** the social services department did not have the power to make the decision;

- **unfair:** the decision was reached in a procedurally unfair manner, or by abuse of power;

- **unreasonable:** all relevant matters were not considered, the law was not properly applied, or there was insufficient consultation.

Human Rights Act 1998

The Human Rights Act 1998 came into force in 2000 and incorporates into English law most of the provisions of the European Convention on Human Rights. The Act applies to all authorities undertaking functions of a public nature, including all care providers in the public sector. The Human Rights Act supports the protection and improvement of the health and welfare of children and young people throughout the United Kingdom. **Article 3** concerns freedom from torture and inhuman or degrading treatment. Children and young people who have been subjected to restraint, seclusion or detention as a result of alarming behaviour could use this part of the Act to raise complaints.

Article 5 concerns the right to liberty and, together with Article 6 concerning the right to a fair hearing, is important for children and young people detained under a section of the Mental Health Act, the Children Act, or within the youth justice system. Social workers involved in such work must ensure that detention is based on sound opinion, in accordance with clearly laid out legal procedures accessible to the individual, and only lasts for as long as the mental health problem persists. In the context of youth justice work, particular attention needs to be paid to the quality and tone of pre-sentence reports which can be stigmatising. The formulaic structure of pre-sentence reports might not enable an assessing social worker working under deadline pressure to provide an accurate picture of a young person.

Article 8 guarantees the right to privacy and family life. Refugees and asylum-seeking families can become entangled in complex legal procedures relating to citizenship and entitlement. This provision can be invoked when UK authorities are considering whether a person should be deported or remain in this country. Compassionate grounds can be used for children affected by the proposed deportation of a parent or in cases where a parent is not admitted. Social workers attuned to the attachment relationships of often small children can use this knowledge to support Article 8 proceedings. In such circumstances the maintenance of the family unit is paramount.

Workers involved in care proceedings or adoption work will have to consider very carefully whether such plans are in the best interests of the child but also are consistent with the child's rights under the Convention. For example, the Convention emphasises that care orders should be a temporary measure and that children should be reunited with their family as soon as possible, where appropriate. In the case of a parent with a mental health problem detained in a psychiatric hospital, the Convention could be employed by their children to facilitate regular visits if these have been denied.

Article 10 concerns basic rights to freedom of expression, and in the context of children's mental health is a crucial safeguard to ensuring that practitioners work actively to enable children and young people to express their opinions about service provision. Workers have an opportunity within this specific provision to articulate and put into practice their value principles of partnership and children's rights.

Article 14 states that all children have an equal claim to the rights set out in the Convention *'irrespective of the child's or his or her parent's or legal guardian's race, colour, sex, language, religion, political or other opinion, national, ethnic or social origin, property, disability, birth or other status'*. This provision could be used to argue for equality of service provision and non-prejudicial diagnosis or treatment. Workers need to ensure they are employing anti-racist and non-discriminatory practice as well as facilitating children and young people to:

- access information about their rights;

- contact mental health services;

- access advocates and children's rights organisations;

- create children's service user groups.

What is your role in CAMHS?

Staff in a variety of work contexts in statutory or voluntary agencies, organised generically or in specialist teams, wherever they are likely to encounter children and young people as clients or carers, are potentially going to need to develop awareness and skills in child and adolescent mental health practice.

✎ Activity 7.3

🔦 Refer to the previously presented material and consider the ways in which the legal and organisational framework affects your role in child and adolescent mental health.

⌨ Commentary

In terms of the policy and organisational context, advice from the Children's Legal Centre is that workers need to follow these principles when planning to intervene in the lives of children and young people on the grounds of disturbed or disturbing behaviour.

- **Informing** the child fully, consulting the child and taking their views and wishes into consideration.

- **Accepting** that in the absence of any specific statutory limitation, children gain the right to make decisions for themselves when they have 'sufficient understanding and intelligence'.

- **Respecting** in particular the child's independent right to consent or withhold consent to treatment as appropriate; and where a child is incapable of giving an informed consent ensuring that the parents' consent is sought, save in emergencies.

- **Ensuring** that any intervention is the least restrictive alternative, and leads to the least possible segregation from the child's family, friends, community and ordinary school.

- **Accessing** independent visitors, advice and advocacy organisations should be available to children who do not have the support of family or friends when it comes to their treatment decisions. In the event of a parent wishing to override the child's refusal to be treated, a legal challenge may be justified if there is evidence that the parent is not acting in the best interests of the child.

A great deal of work will however involve delivering or commissioning family support work linked to formal or informal assessment procedures designed to find out the best way of intervening to prevent children being removed from the care of their parents or deprived of their liberty. The signs and symptoms of mental health problems may not manifest clearly, or even if they do, alternative and sometimes punitive explanations for a young person's behaviour may obscure an underlying psychological problem.

It is important to locate your role in this area of practice in its wider policy and professional context. A useful way of doing this is to consider in general terms what your role is in relation to other professionals working with children and families.

Collaborative or partnership working are terms used frequently in the practice guidance and professional literature without a great deal of reflection about what the terms mean or how to realise them in practice. The concepts need to be embedded within inter-agency child and adolescent mental health working. This ensures that professionals are working together to agree a shared outcome for the child or young person and their family by having a common focus and by helping to support the child with the results they need for optimum psychological development and well-being. Many inquiries have cited the lack of co-operation and communication across professionals and agencies as the reason why children have been harmed or killed by parents or carers.

Communication is important not only to support and develop relationships with families, but also to be able to work well with other professionals. Clients have concerns about the standard of communication they receive and it is the professional's responsibility to ensure it improves and to acknowledge that the families personally need information throughout your contact with them.

Traditionally, health services have tended to focus their attention on a particular problem. For example, psychiatric services focus on mental health, drug and alcohol services on drug and alcohol abuse, and paediatric services on physical health. CAMHS guidelines often concentrate on the management of a single mental disorder instead of taking a holistic and co-ordinated approach to care and treatment of the whole person. Too often young people complain that specialist CAMH services focus on their symptoms or diagnostic label and ignore their social needs.

This narrow approach, however, does not reflect the complexity of health problems experienced by children and adolescents, as young people with mental health problems in one area often experience difficulties in other areas of their lives.

Physical problems may be a consequence of mental health problems while emotional well-being can be adversely affected by a physical illness. Individual professions and services must pay more attention to the high levels of multiple problems in young people, and they need to develop strong collaborative relationships with each other if they are to provide adolescents with effective help for their problems. For example, a young person with depression may very well also have drug and alcohol problems and ADHD. This is where you can make a big contribution to a troubled young person's emotional well-being by taking a whole-person holistic view of their experiences and circumstances.

⚔ Summary of key points

✦ The legal framework for CAMHS encompasses juvenile justice, human rights, mental health, education and social services law. The issues of client consent and confidentiality are especially important in the context of children's rights principles. The link between child mental health and child abuse highlights the crucial role workers have in understanding the legal contexts for informing assessment and intervention.

✦ Children without the support of family or friends in treatment decisions should have access to independent visitors, advice and advocacy organisations. In the event of a parent wishing to override the child's refusal to be treated, a legal challenge may be justified if there is evidence that the parent is not acting in the best interests of the child.

✦ Collaborative or partnership working are terms used frequently in the practice guidance and professional literature without a great deal of reflection about what the terms mean or how to realise them in practice.

✦ Communication is important not only to support and develop relationships with families, but also to be able to work well with other professionals. Clients have concerns about the standard of communication they receive and it is the professional's responsibility to ensure it improves and acknowledge that the families personally need information throughout your contact with them.

Further reading

Children's Rights Alliance for England (2012) *Children's Human Rights: What They Are and Why They Matter*. London: Children's Rights Alliance for England.

Coram Voice (2017) *Advocacy: A Guide for Professionals*. London: Coram Voice.

Department of Health/National Institute for Mental Health in England (2009) *The Legal Aspects of the Care and Treatment of Children and Young People with Mental Disorder: A Guide for Professionals*. London: DH.

Jones, P (ed) (2011) *Children's Rights in Practice*. London: Sage.

Marshall, L and Smith, N (2017) *Supporting Mental Health in Schools and Colleges*. London: National Centre for Social Research.

NHS England (2014) *Model Child and Adolescent Mental Health Specification for Targeted and Specialist Services (Tiers 2/3)*. London: NHS England.

Internet resources

Children's Legal Centre: **www.childrenslegalcentre.com**

Outreach Youth: **www.outreachyouth.org.uk**

Schools resources: **www.mentallyhealthyschools.org.uk**

REFERENCES

Action for Children (nd) The Sooner the Better: Spotting the Signs of Mental Health Issues in Your Child and What to Do to Help. [online] Available at: www.actionforchildren.org.uk/support-for-parents/children-s-mental-health (accessed 20 February 2019).

Banaschewski, T, Zuddas, A, Asherson, P, Buitelaar, J, Coghill, D, Danckaerts, M, Döpfner, M, Rohde, L A, Sonuga-Barke, E and Taylor, E (2015) *ADHD and Hyperkinetic Disorder*, 2nd edn. Oxford: Oxford Psychiatry Library.

Bhui, K and McKenzie, K (2008) Rates and Risk Factors by Ethnic Group for Suicides within a Year of Contact with Mental Health Services in England and Wales. *Psychiatric Services*, 59(4): 414–20.

Bird, L and Falkener, A (2000) *Suicide and Self-Harm*. London, Mental Health Foundation.

Campbell, S, Morley, D and Catchpole, R (eds) (2016) *Critical Issues in Child and Adolescent Mental Health*. London, Palgrave Macmillan.

Care Quality Commission (CQC) (2013) Report Warns of Need for Continued Vigilance and Monitoring of Controlled Drugs. [online] Available at: www.cqc.org.uk/news/releases/report-warns-need-continued-vigilance-monitoring-controlled-drugs (accessed 20 February 2019).

Care Quality Commission (CQC) (2018) *Review of Children and Young People's Mental Health Services: Phase One Report*. London: Care Quality Commission.

Children's Commissioner (2018) *Children's Mental Health Briefing*. London: Children's Commissioner.

Department for Education (2018) Statistics: Looked-After Children. [online] Available at: www.gov.uk/government/collections/statistics-looked-after-children (accessed 20 February 2019).

Department of Health and Social Care (DHSC) (2017) *Transforming Children and Young People's Mental Health Provision: A Green Paper*. London: DHSC.

Doherty, B, Charman, T, Johnson, M H, Scerif, G and Gliga, T (2016) Visual Search and Autism Symptoms. *Developmental Science*, 21(5). doi:10.1111./desc 12661.

Emerson, E and Hatton, C (2007) The Mental Health of Children and Adolescents with Learning Disabilities in Britain. *Advances in Mental Health and Learning Disabilities*, 1(3): 62–3. https://doi.org/10.1108/17530180200700033.

Frances, A J (2011) The British Psychological Society Condemns DSM 5. *Psychology Today*. [online] Available at: www.psychologytoday.com/gb/blog/dsm5-in-distress/201107/the-british-psychological-society-condemns-dsm-5 (accessed 20 February 2019).

Freer, M (2016) *The Mental Health Consultation with a Young Person*. London: Royal College of General Practitioners.

Gohilipour, B (2013) *Grandparents and Grandchildren Can Protect Each Other's Mental Health*. Bath: Live Science.

The Guardian (20 October 2017a) Children Waiting up to 18 Months for Mental Health Treatment – CQC. [online] Available at www.theguardian.com/society/2017/oct/20/children-waiting-up-to-18-months-for-mental-health-treatment-cqc (accessed 20 February 2019).

The Guardian (10 October 2017b) School Exclusions Data in England 'Only the Tip of the Iceberg'. [online] Available at www.theguardian.com/education/2017/oct/10/school-exclusion-figures-date-england-only-tip-iceberg (accessed 20 February 2019).

The Guardian (14 May 2018) Mental Health Referrals in English Schools Rise Sharply. [online] Available at: www.theguardian.com/society/2018/may/14/mental-health-referrals-in-english-schools-rise-sharply-nspcc (accessed 11 February 2019).

Her Majesty's Inspectorate of Prisons (2017) HM Chief Inspector of Prisons Annual Report: 2016 to 2017. [online] Available at: www.gov.uk/government/publications/hm-chief-inspector-of-prisons-annual-report-2016-to-2017 (accessed 20 February 2019).

House of Lords (2018) Youth Services. [online] Available at: https://hansard.parliament.uk/lords/2018-06-26/debates/928B4E3B-9D8B-40DC-9CA1-C02984A37AD0/YouthServices (accessed 20 February 2019).

Human Rights Act (1998) House of Commons, London: HMSO.

Institute of Fiscal Studies (2011) Child and Working-Age Poverty from 2010 to 2020. [online] Available at: www.ifs.org.uk/publications/5711 (accessed 20 February 2019).

Laye-Gindhu, A and Schonert-Reichl, K A (2005) Nonsuicidal Self-Harm Among Community Adolescents: Understanding the 'Whats' and 'Whys' of Self-Harm, *Journal of Youth and Adolescence*, 34(5): 447–57. https://doi:10.1007/s10964-005-7262-z.

Mindfulness Institute (nd) Teacher Training. [online] Available at: www.themindfulness initiative.org.uk/about-mindfulness/teacher-training (accessed 20 February 2019).

Morgan, C, Webb, R T, Carr, M J, Kontopantelis, E, Green, J, Chew-Graham, C A, Kapur, N and Ashcroft, D M (2017) Incidence, Clinical Management, and Mortality Risk Following Self Harm among Children and Adolescents: Cohort Study in Primary Care. *British Medical Journal*, 359. https://doi.org/10.1136/bmj.j4351.

NatCen (2017) British Social Attitudes. [online] Available at: www.natcen.ac.uk/our-research/research/british-social-attitudes (accessed 20 February 2019).

National Autistic Society (nd) Autism Facts and History. [online] Available at: www.autism.org.uk/about/what-is/myths-facts-stats.aspx (accessed 20 February 2019).

National Institute for Clinical Excellence (NICE) (2017) *Eating Disorders: Recognition and Treatment*. London, NICE.

Nuffield Trust (2018) Hospital Admissions as a Result of Self-Harm in Children and Young People. [online] Available at: www.nuffieldtrust.org.uk/resource/hospital-admissions-as-a-result-of-self-harm-in-children-and-young-people (accessed 20 February 2019).

O'Brien, D, Harvey, K, Reardon, T and Cresswell, C (2017) *GPs' Experiences of Children with Anxiety Disorders in Primary Care: A Qualitative Study. British Journal of General Practice*, 67(665): 888–98.

Office for National Statistics (ONS) (2017) *Suicides in the UK: 2017 Registrations*. London: Office for National Statistics.

Pitchforth, J, Fahy, K, Ford, T, Wolpert, M, Viner, R M and Hargreaves, D S (2018) Mental Health and Well-being Trends among Children and Young People in the UK, 1995–2014: Analysis of Repeated Cross-sectional National Health Surveys. *Psychological Medicine*. https://doi.org/10.1017/S0033291718001757.

Punja, S, Shamseer, L, Hartling, L, Urichuk, L, Vandermeer, B, Nikles, J and Vohra, S (2016) Amphetamines for Attention Deficit Hyperactivity Disorder in Children and Adolescents. *Cochrane*. [online] Available at: www.cochrane.org/CD009996/BEHAV_amphetamines-attention-deficit-hyperactivity-disorder-children-and-adolescents (accessed 20 February 2019).

Refugee Council (2018) Children in the Asylum System. [online] Available at: www.refugeecouncil.org.uk/assets/0004/4610/Children_in_the_Asylum_System_Nov_2018.pdf (accessed 20 February 2019).

Rodway, C, Tham, G, Saied, I, Turnbull, P, Windfhur, K, Shaw, J, Kapur, N and Appleby, L (2016) Suicide in Children and Young People in England: A Consecutive Case Series. *The Lancet*, 3(8): 751–9.

Royal College of GPs (2017) BMA Survey Results Are a Call for Help, says RCGP Chair. [online] Available at: www.rcgp.org.uk/about-us/news/2017/september/bma-survey-results-a-call-for-help-says-rcgp-chair.aspx (accessed 20 February 2019).

Rutter, M, Bishop, D, Pine, D, Scott, S, Stephenson, J, Taylor, E and Thapar, A (2008) *Rutter's Child and Adolescent Psychiatry*, 5th edn. London: Blackwell.

Sette, G, Copolla, G and Rosalinda, C (2015) The Transmission of Attachment across Generations: The State of Art and New Theoretical Perspectives. *Scandinavian Journal of Psychology*, 56(3): 315–26.

Unicef (nd) Convention on the Rights of the Child. [online] Available at: www.unicef.org/crc (accessed 20 February 2019).

Walker, S (2010) Young People's Mental Health: The Spiritual Power of Fairy Stories, Myths and Legends. *Mental Health, Religion & Culture*, 13(1): 81–94.

Walker, S (2011a) *The Social Worker's Guide to Child and Adolescent Mental Health*. London: Jessica Kingsley.

Walker, S (2011b) Cyber Bullying and the Impact on Young People's Mental Health. *Young Minds*, Winter 2011/12: 18–114.

Walker, S (2012a) *Responding to Self-Harm in Children and Adolescents: A Professional's Guide to Treatment, Identification and Support*. London: Jessica Kingsley.

Walker, S (2012b) The Effects of Cyber-Bullying on the Mental Health of Young People. Scientific Paper Presentation to the 7th International Conference on Interdisciplinary Social Sciences, Barcelona.

Walker, S (2016) Cultural Context and Socially Inclusive Practice. In Campbell, S, Morley, D and Catchpole, R (eds) *Critical Issues in Child and Adolescent Mental Health* (pp 101–18). London: Palgrave Macmillan.

INDEX

characteristics, 10

characteristics of, 59–60

diagnosis, 10–11

gender differences in, 60

supporting goals, 60–1

symptoms, 11

autonomy, 43

behaviour well-being, impact of food
and diet on, 36–7

belonging, sense of, 64–7

bipolar disorder, recommended
treatments for, 82

Black, 49

access to help, 53

history of childhood mental health
problems, 69

and racism, 52

understanding of families of, 49–50

Bowlby's attachment theory, 25

breathing exercise, 90

brief family work, 102–3

British Psychological Society, 124

British Social Attitudes (BSA), 108, 110

bulimia nervosa, 13–14

recommended treatments, 82

Care Quality Commission (CQC), 1

challenging ability, 68

child and adolescent development, 24

Bowlby's attachment theory, 25

Eriksen's psycho-social stages of
development, 25–6

Freud's psychosexual stages of
development, 24

needs, 32

personality development, 26–7

Piaget's stages of cognitive
development, 26

sociology, 27–8

Child and Adolescent Mental Health
Services (CAMHS), 1, 2, 8, 22,
56–7, 62, 63, 83, 115, 127, 138,
148, 150–2

child development centres, 56

child poverty, 114

child-centred planning, for learning
difficulties, 57

childhood, understanding of, 27–8

Children Act 1989, 13, 111, 140,
145–6

definition of disability in, 146–7

on professional practice, 148

Children and Young People's Mental
Health and Wellbeing
Taskforce, 137

Children's Legal Centre, 139

children's rights. See rights, of
young people

circular questioning, 101–2

cognitive behavioural practice, 85

Common Assessment Framework, 146

common, definition of, 5

safety, parenting capacity, 32

schizophrenia, 14–16

    intervention's outcome, 15–16

    recommended treatments, 82

    risk factors, 15

    signs, 14

    treatment and management of, 15

schools

    exclusions, 39–40, 63

    future role of, 115

    phobia, 10

secured attachment, 42

self-care skills, child's developmental need, 32

self-efficacy, 44

self-esteem, 43, 44

    cyber-bullying's impact on, 122

self-harm, 1, 12. *See also* suicide

    assessment of, 117–19

    coping mechanism, 118–19

    as coping method, 119

    definition of, 8, 115–16

    family's role in, 116–17

    prevalence, 116–17

    recommended treatments, 82

    sustaining support, 119–20

self-respect, 36

separation anxiety disorder, 9–10

sexual abuse, 37, 40, 94

sexual issues, 96–7, 114

sexual orientation, 131–2

sin, sense of, 54

sociability, 43

social dimension affecting children's mental health, 21

social entrepreneurship, 67

social exclusion, 64

social inclusion, 67–8

    of children and adolescent with learning difficulties, 58

social media, 96, 118, 121

social networking, and cyberbullying, 122, 123

social presentation, child's developmental need, 32

social relationships

    child's developmental need, 32

socio-economic status, 23, 99

solution-focused model, 102–3

Special Educational Needs and Disability Act 2001, 140

special needs educational services, 56

specialist LD services, 56

spirituality, 50

    importance of, 53–4

stability, parenting capacity, 33

stimulation, parenting capacity, 32

Strengths and Difficulties Questionnaire (SDQ), 34

strengths and difficulties, appreciation of, 33–4

Other books you may be interested in:

Active Social Work with Children with Disabilities
By Julie Adams and Diana Leshone

ISBN 978-1-910391-94-5

Observing Children and Families: Beyond the Surface
By Gill Butler

ISBN 978-1-910391-62-4

Psychosocial and Relationship-based Practice
By Claudia Megele

ISBN 978-1-909682-97-9

The Critical Years: Child Development from Conception to Five
By Tim Gully

ISBN 978-1-909330-73-3

The W Word: Witchcraft Labelling and Child Safeguarding
in Social Work Practice
By Prospera Tedam and Awura Adjoa

ISBN 978-1-912096-00-8

Titles are also available in a range of electronic formats. To order please go to our website www.criticalpublishing.com or contact our distributor NBN International, 10 Thornbury Road, Plymouth PL6 7PP, telephone 01752 202301 or email orders@ nbninternational.com